Adult Congenital Heart Disease

Editors

SAURABH RAJPAL
RAGAVENDRA R. BALIGA

HEART FAILURE CLINICS

www.heartfailure.theclinics.com

Consulting Editor
EDUARDO BOSSONE

Founding Editor
JAGAT NARULA

April 2024 • Volume 20 • Number 2

ELSEVIER

1600 John F. Kennedy Boulevard • Suite 1800 • Philadelphia, Pennsylvania, 19103-2899

http://www.theclinics.com

HEART FAILURE CLINICS Volume 20, Number 2
April 2024 ISSN 1551-7136, ISBN-13: 978-0-443-13151-6

Editor: Joanna Gascoine
Developmental Editor: Nitesh Barthwal

Heart Failure Clinics (ISSN 1551-7136) is published quarterly by Elsevier Inc., 360 Park Avenue South, New York, NY 10010-1710. Months of publication are January, April, July, and October. Business and editorial offices: 1600 John F. Kennedy Boulevard, Suite 1800, Philadelphia, PA 19103-2899. Periodicals postage paid at New York, NY, and additional mailing offices. Subscription prices are USD 297.00 per year for US individuals, USD 100.00 per year for US students and residents, USD 324.00 per year for Canadian individuals, USD 341.00 per year for international individuals, and USD 100.00 per year for Canadian and foreign students/residents. For institutional access pricing please contact Customer Service via the contact information below. To receive student and resident rate, orders must be accompanied by name of affiliated institution, date of term, and the *signature* of program/residency coordinator on institution letterhead. Orders will be billed at individual rate until proof of status is received. Foreign air speed delivery is included in all *Clinics* subscription prices. All prices are subject to change without notice. **POSTMASTER:** Send address changes to *Heart Failure Clinics*, Elsevier Health Sciences Division, Subscription Customer Service, 3251 Riverport Lane, Maryland Heights, MO 63043. **Customer Service: 1-800-654-2452 (US and Canada). From outside of the US and Canada, call 314-447-8871. Fax: 314-447-8029. For print support, E-mail: JournalsCustomerService-usa@elsevier.com. For online support, E-mail: JournalsOnlineSupport-usa@elsevier.com.**

Reprints. For copies of 100 or more of articles in this publication, please contact the Commercial Reprints Department, Elsevier Inc., 360 Park Avenue South, New York, NY 10010-1710. Tel.: 212-633-3874; Fax: 212-633-3820; E-mail: reprints@elsevier.com.

Heart Failure Clinics is covered in *MEDLINE/PubMed (Index Medicus)*.

Contributors

CONSULTING EDITOR

EDUARDO BOSSONE, MD, PhD, FCCP, FESC, FACC
Consulting Editor, *Heart Failure Clinics*, Director of Cardiology, Cardarelli Hospital, Department of Public Health, UNESCO Chair of Health Education and Sustainable Development, Department of Translational Medical Sciences, University of Naples "Federico II," Naples, Italy

EDITORS

SAURABH RAJPAL, MBBS, MD, FACC, FSCMR
Associate Professor, Associate Program Director, Columbus Ohio Adult Congenital Heart Program (COACH), Division of Cardiology, Department of Internal Medicine, The Ohio State University Wexner Medical Center and Nationwide Children's Hospital, Columbus, Ohio, USA

RAGAVENDRA R. BALIGA, MBBS, MD, MBA, FACC, FRCP, FI-CO
Professor, Inaugural Cardio-Oncologist, Cardio-Oncology Center of Excellence; Division of Cardiology, Department of Internal Medicine, The Ohio State University Wexner Medical Center, Columbus, Ohio, USA

EDUARDO BOSSONE, MD, PhD, FCCP, FESC, FACC
Consulting Editor, *Heart Failure Clinics*, Director of Cardiology, Cardarelli Hospital, Department of Public Health, UNESCO Chair of Health Education and Sustainable Development, Department of Translational Medical Sciences, University of Naples "Federico II," Naples, Italy

AUTHORS

GUILLERMO AGORRODY, MD
Fellow, Toronto ACHD Program, Division of Cardiology, Department of Medicine, Peter Munk Cardiac Centre, Toronto General Hospital, University Health Network, University of Toronto, Toronto, Ontario, Canada

NAEL ALDWEIB, MD
Assistant Professor, Knight Institute Oregon Health and Science University, Portland, Oregon, USA

RAFAEL ALONSO-GONZALEZ, MD, MSc, FESC
Director, Toronto ACHD Program, Division of Cardiology, Department of Medicine, Peter Munk Cardiac Centre, Toronto General Hospital, University Health Network, University of Toronto, Toronto, Ontario, Canada

LAITH ALSHAWABKEH, MD, MSCI, FACC, FPICS
Associate Clinical Professor, Adult Congenital Heart Disease Program, Division of Cardiovascular Medicine, Department of Medicine, University of California, San Diego, La Jolla, California, USA

JUDITH BOUCHARDY, MD
Consultant, Department of Cardiology, Hôpitaux Universitaires de Genève, Geneva, Switzerland

CRAIG BROBERG, MD, MS
Professor of Medicine and Radiology, Director of Adult Congenital Heart Disease, Knight Cardiovascular Institute Oregon Health and Science University, Portland, Oregon, USA

ANDREW COLETTI, MD, FACC
Director, Center for Advanced Heart Disease and Transplantation, Providence Spokane Heart Institute, Spokane, Washington, USA

HEIDI M. CONNOLLY, MD
Cardiologist, Department of Cardiovascular Medicine, Mayo Clinic, Rochester, Minnesota, USA

CURT J. DANIELS, MD
Dottie Dohan Shepard Professor in Cardiovascular Medicine, Director, Columbus Ohio Adult Congenital Heart Program (COACH); Professor, Department of Internal Medicine and Pediatrics, The Ohio State University and Nationwide Children's Hospital, Columbus, Ohio, USA

ANUDEEP K. DODEJA, MD
Pediatric and ACHD Cardiologist, Department of Pediatrics, Connecticut Children's, University of Connecticut School of Medicine, Hartford, Connecticut, USA

VALERIA E. DUARTE, MD, MPH
Adult Congenital Cardiologist, Department of Cardiology, Houston Methodist DeBakey Heart and Vascular Center, Houston, Texas, USA

ALEXANDER C. EGBE, MD, MPH, MS, FACC
Professor of Medicine, Department of Cardiovascular Medicine, Mayo Clinic and Foundation, Rochester, Minnesota, USA

NICOLE HERRICK, MD
Resident Physician, Division of Cardiovascular Medicine, Department of Medicine, University of California San Francisco, San Diego, La Jolla, California, USA

RICHARD A. KRASUSKI, MD
Director of Adult Congenital Heart Services, Department of Cardiovascular Medicine, Duke University Medical Center, Durham, North Carolina, USA

JONATHAN KUSNER, MD
Senior Assistant Resident, Department of Medicine, Duke University Medical Center, Durham, North Carolina, USA

MAGALIE LADOUCEUR, MD, PhD
Consultant, Department of Cardiology, Hôpitaux Universitaires de Genève, Geneva, Switzerland; Centre de Recherche Cardiovasculaire de Paris, INSERM U970, Paris, France

MICHAEL J. LANDZBERG, MD
Associated Professor of Medicine, Staff, Boston Adult Congenital Heart (BACH) Group, Heart Pal Team; Department of Cardiology, Brigham and Women's Hospital, Boston Children's Hospital, Harvard Medical School, Department of Psychosocial Oncology and Palliative Care, Dana Farber Cancer Institute, Boston, Massachusetts, USA

WILLIAM H. MARSHALL V, MD
Adult Congenital Heart Disease Cardiologist, Department of Internal Medicine, Division of Cardiovascular Medicine, Davis Heart and Lung Research Institute, Wexner Medical Center at The Ohio State University; The Heart Center, Nationwide Children's Hospital, Columbus, Ohio, USA

PATRICK McCONNELL, MD
Department of Cardiothoracic Surgery, Nationwide Children's Hospital, The Heart Center; Surgical Director, Department of Surgery, Division of Cardiac Surgery, The Ohio State University, Columbus, Ohio, USA

JAMES MUDD, MD
Cardiologist, Center for Advanced Heart Disease and Transplantation, Providence Spokane Heart Institute, Spokane, Washington, USA

JEREMY NICOLARSEN, MD, FACC
Director, Providence Adult and Teen Congenital Heart Program (PATCH), Spokane, Washington, USA

ALEXANDER R. OPOTOWSKY, MD, MMSc
Director, Cincinnati Adult Congenital Heart Disease Program, Professor, Department of Pediatrics, Heart Institute, Cincinnati Children's Hospital, University of Cincinnati College of Medicine, Cincinnati, Ohio, USA

SAURABH RAJPAL, MBBS, MD, FACC, FSCMR
Associate Professor, Associate Program Director, Columbus Ohio Adult Congenital Heart Program (COACH), Division of Cardiology, Department of Internal Medicine, The Ohio State University Wexner Medical Center and Nationwide Children's Hospital, Columbus, Ohio, USA

SHAILENDRA UPADHYAY, MD
Division Head, Department of Pediatric Cardiology, Connecticut Children's, University of Connecticut School of Medicine, Hartford, Connecticut, USA

MARCUS UREY, MD
Associate Clinical Professor, Division of Cardiovascular Medicine, Department of Medicine, University of California San Francisco, San Diego, La Jolla, California, USA

Contents

Adults with congenital heart disease (ACHD) are facing lifelong complications, notably heart failure (HF). This review focuses on classifications, incidence, prevalence, and mortality of HF related to ACHD. Diagnosing HF in ACHD is intricate due to anatomic variations, necessitating comprehensive clinical evaluations. Hospitalizations and resource consumption for ACHD HF have significantly risen compared with non-ACHD HF patients. With more than 30% prevalence in complex cases, HF has become the leading cause of death in ACHD. These alarming trends underscore the insufficient understanding of ACHD-related HF manifestations and management challenges within the context of aging, complexity, and comorbidity.

There is an increasing prevalence of heart failure among the growing, aging population of adults with congenital heart disease (CHD). Direct extrapolation to adults with CHD of standard heart failure definitions and management guidelines developed for adults with acquired forms of heart failure can be problematic. A nuanced and flexible application of clinical judgment founded on a deep understanding of underlying pathophysiology is needed to most effectively leverage the many recent advances in managing acquired heart failure for the care of adults with CHD.

Heart failure (HF) in adult congenital heart disease (ACHD) is an increasingly common problem facing ACHD and advanced heart disease and transplant providers. Patients are highly nuanced, and therapies are poorly studied. Standard HF medications are often used in patients who are not targets of large clinical trials. HF management in this data-free zone requires focused, comprehensive team-based care and close follow-up and communication with patients.

Heart failure (HF) is common in adults with congenital heart disease (CHD), and it is the leading cause of death in this population. Adults with CHD presenting with stage D HF have a poor prognosis, and early recognition of signs of advanced HF and referral for advanced therapies for HF offer the best survival as compared with other therapies. The indications for advanced therapies for HF outlined in this article should serve as a guide for clinicians to determine the optimal time for referral. Palliative care should be part of the multidisciplinary care model for HF in patients with CHD.

complications due to prior surgical interventions, including sternal reentry, collateral vessels, and the neo-aortic root after the Damus–Kaye–Stansel procedure. Surgical considerations for systemic atrioventricular valvular surgery, Fontan revision, and advanced heart failure therapies including ventricular assist devices, heart transplant, and combined heart–liver transplant are discussed, with a focus on unique patient populations including those with systemic right ventricles and those with Fontan circulation.

Already a challenging condition to define, adult congenital heart disease (ACHD) -associated heart failure (HF) often incorporates specific anatomies, including intracardiac and extracardiac shunts, which require rigorous diagnostic characterization and heighten the importance of clinicians proactively considering overall hemodynamic impacts of using specific therapies. The presence of elevated pulmonary vascular resistance dramatically increases the complexity of managing patients with ACHD-HF. Total circulatory management in patients with ACHD-HF requires input from multidisciplinary care teams and thoughtful and careful utilization of medical, interventional, and surgical approaches.

Heart failure in cyanotic congenital heart disease (CHD) is diagnosed clinically rather than relying solely on ventricular function assessments. Patients with cyanosis often present with clinical features indicative of heart failure. Although myocardial injury and dysfunction likely contribute to cyanotic CHD, the primary concern is the reduced delivery of oxygen to tissues. Symptoms such as fatigue, lassitude, dyspnea, headaches, myalgias, and a cold sensation underscore inadequate tissue oxygen delivery, forming the basis for defining heart failure in cyanotic CHD. Thus, it is pertinent to delve into the components of oxygen delivery in this context.

The practice of palliative care (PC) strives to mitigate patient suffering through aligning patient priorities and values with care planning and via improved understanding of complex physical, psychosocial, and spiritual stressors and dynamics that contribute to patient-centered outcomes. Through representative 'case examples' and supportive data, the role and value of a PC consultant, within the framework of a comprehensive adult congenital heart disease (ACHD) team caring for ACHD with advanced heart disease, are reviewed.

HEART FAILURE CLINICS

SERIES OF RELATED INTEREST

Cardiology Clinics
http://www.cardiology.theclinics.com/
Cardiac Electrophysiology Clinics
https://www.cardiacep.theclinics.com/
Interventional Cardiology Clinics
https://www.interventional.theclinics.com/

THE CLINICS ARE AVAILABLE ONLINE!
Access your subscription at:
www.theclinics.com

Preface

Heart Failure in Adults with Congenital Heart Disease: The Time to Act is Now

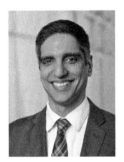

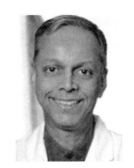

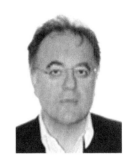

Saurabh Rajpal, MBBS, MD, FACC, FSCMR

Ragavendra R. Baliga, MBBS, MD, MBA, FACC, FRCP, FI-CO

Eduardo Bossone, MD, PhD

Editors

The aim of this work is to provide a comprehensive review of all aspects of heart failure in adults with congenital heart disease (ACHD) (**Fig. 1**). While the surge in heart failure due to acquired heart disease is well-known, the parallel increase in heart failure cases within the congenital heart disease (CHD) population remains underappreciated. Notably, ACHD heart failure is characterized by prolonged hospitalization periods and elevated health care costs compared with acquired heart disease–related heart failure. There is a lack of understanding, not only of the scope of the problem but also of the pathophysiology, diagnosis, and management, as several aspects of heart failure are unique to the ACHD population. This clinically focused compendium, therefore, endeavors to demystify ACHD-related heart failure, providing information on all facets of adult CHD heart failure, including epidemiology, pathophysiology, medical therapy, arrhythmia management, surgical considerations, transplant and mechanical circulatory support, and palliative care. We have also included sections on cardiovascular imaging in ACHD heart failure and caring for specialized populations, such as those with pulmonary hypertension and unrepaired cyanotic heart disease.

CHD is the most prevalent birth defect, a fact that can sometimes elude practitioners focused on adult cardiology, leading to the misconception that CHD is primarily a pediatric concern. Over the past few decades, there have been significant advancements in congenital cardiac surgery, pediatric cardiology, and pediatric intensive cardiac care, leading to increased survival rates among children with even the most complex CHD. Consequently, the landscape of CHD has undergone significant transformation since the early 2000s, resulting in a substantial and increasing number of adult patients with CHD, surpassing the number of children with the condition.

Heart Failure Clin 20 (2024) xi–xii
https://doi.org/10.1016/j.hfc.2024.01.004
1551-7136/24/© 2024 Published by Elsevier Inc.

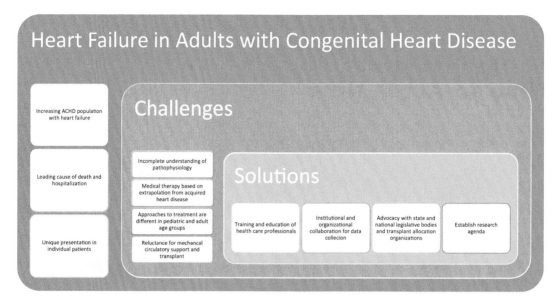

Fig. 1. Heart failure in ACHD.

However, this paradigm shift appears to be accompanied by a perceptual gap among health care professionals in terms of both understanding the scope of the problem and appreciating the unique features of heart failure in each individual patient with ACHD. Key heart failure studies have often excluded individuals with CHD due to perceived complexities, setting a precedent that permeates general practice. Consequently, patients with CHD experience extended waitlist times for transplant consideration and infrequent evaluation as candidates for mechanical circulatory-assist devices. These challenges are compounded by the widening gap in the number of patients with ACHD with heart failure and the availability of teams with the expertise to provide care for these patients. However, a course correction is underway, evident in the expanding indications and exceptions for advanced therapies for heart failure in ACHD.

A significant strength of this issue is that it brings together the efforts of over 15 clinicians in the fields of ACHD and congenital cardiac surgery. It has been an invaluable experience collaborating on this project with subject experts from an international range of institutions. A vision statement and call to action is a one part of this collection to understand the status of the problem for a strategic focus and strive toward alignment of common goals. This collection is intended to serve as a valuable resource for practitioners and researchers seeking the latest insights and best practices in managing heart failure in this unique and ever-increasing population.

DISCLOSURES

S. Rajpal discloses the following: Liquidia Pharmaceuticals, Advisory Board; Medtronic, Travel Fees; Simply Speaking, Speaker Bureau.

Saurabh Rajpal, MBBS, MD, FACC, FSCMR
Division of Cardiology
Department of Internal Medicine
The Ohio State University
Wexner Medical Center
Nationwide Children's Hospital
473 West 12th Avenue
Columbus, OH 43210, USA

Ragavendra R. Baliga, MBBS, MD, MBA, FACC,
FRCP, FI-CO
Cardio-Oncology Center of Excellence
Division of Cardiology
Department of Internal Medicine
The Ohio State University
Wexner Medical Center
473 West 12th Avenue
Columbus, OH 43210, USA

Eduardo Bossone, MD, PhD
Department of Public Health
Department of Translational Medical Sciences
University of Naples "Federico II"
Ed. 18, I piano, Via Sergio Pansini 5
Naples 80131, Italy

E-mail addresses:
saurabh.rajpal@osumc.edu (S. Rajpal)
rrbaliga@gmail.com (R.R. Baliga)
eduardo.bossone@unina.it (E. Bossone)

Epidemiology and Definition of Heart Failure in Adult Congenital Heart Disease

Magalie Ladouceur, MD, PhD[a,b,*], Judith Bouchardy, MD[a]

KEYWORDS

• Congenital heart disease • Chronic disease • Heart failure • Prevalence • Risk factor

KEY POINTS

• Diagnosing heart failure (HF) in adult congenital heart disease (ACHD) patients presents challenges because of variations in cardiac anatomy, pathophysiology, and clinical presentation. Various classification systems have been proposed but are yet to be refined to improve the identification of ACHD-related HF. As a result, there is significant variation in the definition of HF among epidemiologic studies related to ACHD HF.

• HF-related hospitalizations have shown a significant increase over the last decades, surpassing the increase in HF hospitalizations in non-ACHD HF, due to the increase in older patients with complex CHD lesions. ACHD HF accounts for 30% of hospitalizations and requires more health resources than non-ACHD-HF cases. ACHD HF is generally more severe than non-ACHD with a higher rate of readmission and a 5-year mortality reaching almost 60%.

• Risk factors for HF in ACHD patients include the underlying cardiac diagnosis, tolerance signs, cardiac function, conventional risk factors, and cardiac comorbidities, all of which require increased attention. Few predictive models have been developed that may aid in identifying ACHD patients at risk of HF, thereby warranting more active management. Further investigation is required to comprehensively assess emerging risk factors and multiomics influences.

INTRODUCTION

The progressive rise in the population of adults with congenital heart disease (ACHD) is a notable occurrence attributable to historical and contemporary advances in cardiac surgery and congenital cardiology domains. It is estimated that an overwhelming 85% to 90% of infants born with congenital heart defects (CHDs) reach adult age. So that the present number of ACHD patients surpasses the number of children with CHD in Western countries. Moreover, predictions suggest that the population of ACHD will experience an approximate 60% surge per decade.[1] This, in turn, triggers a continuous expansion of the ACHD population vulnerable to complications, including heart failure (HF). Indeed, despite the progress that has been made, the vast majority of ACHD patients are not cured and suffer from lifelong complications including arrhythmias, needs for interventions and reoperations, pulmonary hypertension, extracardiac complications, and especially HF. The risk of HF in ACHD patients is high,[2,3] and HF has become the leading cause of death in this cardiac disease.[4,5] The increase in HF-related deaths reported in ACHD presents a compelling impetus to investigate the most current data concerning HF epidemiology. The aim is to elucidate the factors contributing to the enduring

[a] Department of Cardiology, Hôpitaux Universitaires de Genève, Rue Gabrielle-Perret-Gentil 4, Geneva 1211, Switzerland; [b] Centre de Recherche Cardiovasculaire de Paris, INSERM U970, 56 rue Leblanc, Paris 75015, France
* Corresponding author.
E-mail address: magalie.ladouceur@gmail.com

Heart Failure Clin 20 (2024) 113–127
https://doi.org/10.1016/j.hfc.2023.12.001
1551-7136/24/© 2023 Elsevier Inc. All rights reserved.

burden of HF in ACHD. These factors may encompass a rise in incidence, necessitating intensified primary prevention efforts, or deteriorating outcomes, demanding more efficacious treatment and management strategies.

Initially, a comprehensive examination of HFs taxonomy in ACHD will be undertaken to explore how different classifications impact our comprehension of its epidemiology. Subsequently, up-to-date data concerning the incidence, prevalence, mortality, and hospitalization rates of HF related to ACHD will be explored. Furthermore, this review delves into data pertaining to risk factors. By doing so, this review aims to identify gaps in our current knowledge and delineate future avenues for research.

DELINEATION OF HEART FAILURE IN ADULT WITH CONGENITAL HEART DISEASE

As most cardiac diseases reach their advanced stage, it is not surprising that HF emerges as a prominent complication in ACHD patients. When exploring the epidemiology of a disease, it is crucial to establish clear criteria for diagnosing and categorizing its severity. In the case of ACHD-related HF, this pivotal process entails considering the epidemiologic definitions, various HF presentations and stages, including the emerging concept of advanced HF and cardiac function assessments (**Fig. 1**).

Over the years, various HF definitions have been proposed. According to the definition put forth by Poole-Wilson, HF is characterized as a "clinical syndrome resulting from an abnormality of the heart and distinguished by a characteristic pattern of responses involving hemodynamics, renal, neural, and hormonal factors."[6] This comprehensive definition acknowledges the potential multifactorial nature of HF and its independence from sole factors like low cardiac output or depressed systolic ventricular function.

Recognizing and quantifying HF in ACHD patients presents a challenge due to the diverse variations in underlying anatomic substrates. HF occurs when the heart fails to meet the body's metabolic demands, and failure to identify it may result in multiorgan dysfunction, increased morbidity, and mortality. The guidelines strongly emphasize that HF is primarily a clinical diagnosis and should not be solely reliant on a single diagnostic test, a principle that extends to patients with CHD as well.[7-9] Classical signs and symptoms of HF are apparent particularly in older ACHD individuals. However, in younger patients, subclinical HF is common and challenging to detect, as compensatory autonomic and renal adjustments can maintain normal blood pressure and urine output. In addition, individuals who have adapted to chronic heart disease over their lifetime may underreport symptoms.[10] Even though exercise capacity might be reduced, patients could lack typical HF symptoms and signs, even reporting the New York Heart Association (NYHA) functional class I, and patients may not recognize subtle changes in their functional class. As a result, using general HF classifications like the NYHA categories might underestimate disease severity, especially in those with complex or cyanotic CHD. Although the NYHA classification might underestimate the degree of limitation in certain ACHD patients, it remains a valuable clinical instrument. A strong correlation with objective exercise measures, the severity of

ACHD-HF definition : various pathophysiology and clinical presentation
→ Need to refine ACHD-HF criteria and classification
→ Consider at least NYHA to classify HF severity

ACHD-HF incidence
- 1.2‰ to 3.16‰ person-year
- Increase with ACHD complexity (SRV & Fontan) and age (35% of patient > 65-year-old)

ACHD –HF severity
- Leading cause of death
- 60% of 5-year mortality
- Higher rate of early and late readmission

Resource allocation:
Dedicated ACHD-HF clinic
Reduce readmission risk:
- Longer initial hospital stays
- Medical interventions

Fig. 1. Definition and epidemiology of heart failure (HF) related to adult congenital heart disease (ACHD). NYHA FC, the New York Heart Association functional classification; SRV, systemic right ventricle.

underlying cardiac conditions, and mid- to long-term mortality has been recently shown.[11] Therefore, the NYHA should not be disregarded as a means of detection of HF in ACHD. There is inadequate evidence that categorizing patients with CHD by the American Heart Association/American College of Cardiology congestive HF stages system[8] enables management decisions or improves outcome. The recently introduced anatomic and physiologic classification system holds potential for distinguishing ACHD patients who might develop new or exacerbated HF.[12] However, further refinement and investigation are necessary to enhance its ability to identify ACHD individuals at risk of HF. The Seattle Heart Failure Model (SHFM) has been shown to be effective in identifying ACHD patients at risk of adverse outcomes and may have an interesting role in the identification of ACHD-related HF.[13] **Table 1** suggests the different classifications system that can be used in ACHD-related HF.

Consequently, there is a considerable variation in the definitions and consistency criteria for HF in ACHD, meaning that the number of patients suffering from this complication is likely to be underestimated. This is especially evident in CHD with a single ventricle and Fontan circulation failure. In Fontan, systemic venous blood is directly connected to the pulmonary circulation, shunting the single ventricle and creating two circulations in series. This circulation is characterized by an elevation of the central venous pressure, lack of pulsatility in the pulmonary arteries, and low cardiac output. By definition, Fontan (patho)physiology responds to HF criteria from Fontan completion. A "failing Fontan" circulation is an almost inevitable long-term consequence of the altered physiology. Failing Fontan is a nonspecific generic term describing a dysfunction of the Fontan circulation, which can be related to various etiologies (systolic or diastolic single ventricle dysfunction, valvular dysfunction, increased pulmonary vascular resistance, and so forth) and leads to various symptoms such as typical congestive signs but also hypoxemia or impairment of vital organs, including liver disease, protein-losing enteropathy, and plastic bronchitis.[17]

Advanced HF is a significant clinical designation with implications for advanced therapies like transplant and mechanical ventricular support. Professional societies, such as the Heart Failure Society of America, American College of Cardiology/American Heart Association, Heart Failure Association, and European Society of Cardiology, have outlined criteria to characterize this state. Only one study reported incidence and outcome on advanced HF in ACHD using ESC criteria to define advanced HF stage in ACHD.[18]

INCIDENCE, MORTALITY, AND PREVALENCE

These measures are the foundation of epidemiology investigations of the burden of a given disease in populations. The prevalence of HF refers to the number of patients affected by this condition at any given period or throughout their entire life. Calculating the current prevalence is typically straightforward, as cross-sectional studies effectively reveal the proportion of individuals with HF at the time of data collection. Determining the lifetime prevalence of HF is more intricate due to the unavailability of a comprehensive chronologic record of a patient's medical history. In the context of HF related to ACHD, it is logical to consider that documenting an HF diagnosis later in life or at the time of death can act as a valuable proxy for estimating lifetime HF occurrences. This assumption is based on the escalating risk of HF over time in patients with ACHD, as HF manifests as a progressive, persistent condition that is usually not eradicated by interventions (although symptoms may be alleviated). Prevalence also informs resource allocation decisions by providing a valuable perspective on the existing burden of disease.

The incidence of HF refers to the number of new cases that occur within a given period. This calculation typically requires access to continuous data and is therefore more computationally complex than assessing cases of point prevalence. Understanding the incidence of HF across the spectrum of CHD, segmented by age, provides critical information for prospective service planning. Furthermore, analyzing the incidence of HF provides valuable insights into how the occurrence of HF may have evolved over time due to shifts in the characteristics and risk factors of ACHD.

The credibility of these assessments hinges on the use of consistent and standardized criteria, with efforts made to mitigate any undue influence from the incorporation of diagnostic methods that could artificially inflate disease detection rates. Nevertheless, it is essential to acknowledge a notable variability in the definition of ACHD-related HF within research, as discussed earlier. Most recent studies analyzed administrative data that rely on diagnostic codes. As such, they are subject to several biases including shifts in coding. Moreover, estimates of the prevalence/incidence of overt HF unexpectedly underestimate the true prevalence/incidence of HF as it relies on cases coming to medical attention.

The 2023 American Heart Association Statistical Update estimates the prevalence of HF to be 6.7 million and is projected to affect 3% of the US population in 2030.[19] The prevalence increases

Table 1
Classification systems based on 2018 American Heart Association/ American College of Cardiology (AHA/ACC) management of adult congenital heart disease[8,14–16]

NYHA Functional Class	Canadian Cardiovascular Society Grading for Angina Pectoris	Specific Activity Scale	AHA/ACC Stages of HF	Warnes-Somerville Ability Index	Physiologic Stage of ACHD AP Classification
Patients with cardiac disease but without resulting limitations of physical activity. Ordinary physical activity does not cause undue fatigue, palpitation, dyspnea, or anginal pain.	Ordinary physical activity such as walking and climbing stairs does not cause angina. Angina with strenuous or rapid prolonged exertion at work or recreation.	Patients can perform to completion any activity requiring ≥7 metabolic equivalents (eg, can carry 24 lb up 8 steps, do outdoor work [shovel snow, spade soil], and do recreational activities [skiing, basketball, squash, handball, jog/walk 5 mph]).	Patients at high risk of developing HF because of the presence of conditions that is strongly associated with the development of HF. Such patients have no identified structural or functional abnormalities of the pericardium, myocardium, or cardiac valves and have never shown signs or symptoms of HF.	Normal life; full-time work or school; can manage pregnancy.	NYHA class I (No symptoms and no limitation in ordinary physical activity, e.g. shortness of breath when walking, climbing stairs etc)No arrhythmiaNormal exercise capacityNo hemodynamic or anatomic sequelaeNormal renal, hepatic, and pulmonary function
Patients with cardiac disease resulting in slight limitation of physical activity. They are comfortable at rest. Ordinary physical activity results in fatigue, palpitation, dyspnea, or anginal pain.	Slight limitation of ordinary activity. Walking or climbing stairs rapidly; walking uphill; walking or stair climbing after meals, in cold, in wind, or when under emotional stress; or	Patients can perform to completion any activity requiring ≤5 metabolic equivalents (eg, have sexual intercourse without stopping, garden, rake, weed, roller skate, dance fox trot, and walk at	Patients who have developed structural heart disease that is strongly associated with the development of HF but who have never shown signs or symptoms of HF.	Able to do part-time work; life modified by symptoms.	NYHA FC II symptoms Mild hemodynamic sequelae (mild aortic enlargement, mild ventricular enlargement, mild ventricular dysfunction) Mild valvular disease Trivial or small shunt

	only during the few hours after awakening. Walking >2 blocks on level ground and climbing >1 flight of ordinary stairs at a normal pace and in normal conditions.	4 mph on level ground), but cannot and do not perform to completion activities requiring ≥7 metabolic equivalents.			(not hemodynamically significant) Arrhythmia not requiring treatment Abnormal objective cardiac limitation to exercise
Patients with cardiac disease resulting in marked limitation of physical activity. They are comfortable at rest. Less than ordinary physical activity causes fatigue, palpitation, dyspnea, or anginal pain.	Marked limitation of ordinary physical activity. Walking 1–2 blocks on level ground and climbing 1 flight in normal conditions.	Patients can perform to completion any activity requiring ≤2 metabolic equivalents (eg, shower without stopping, strip and make bed, clean windows, walk 2.5 mph, bowl, play golf, and dress without stopping), but cannot and do not perform to completion any activities requiring >5 metabolic equivalents.	Patients who have current or prior symptoms of HF associated with underlying structural heart disease.	Unable to work; noticeable limitation of activities.	NYHA FC III symptoms Significant (moderate or greater) valvular disease; moderate or greater ventricular dysfunction (systemic, pulmonic, or both) Moderate aortic enlargement Venous or arterial stenosis Mild or moderate hypoxemia/cyanosis Hemodynamically significant shunt Arrhythmias controlled with treatment Pulmonary hypertension (less than severe) End-organ dysfunction responsive to therapy

(continued on next page)

Table 1
(continued)

NYHA Functional Class	Canadian Cardiovascular Society Grading for Angina Pectoris	Specific Activity Scale	AHA/ACC Stages of HF	Warnes-Somerville Ability Index	Physiologic Stage of ACHD AP Classification
Patient with cardiac disease resulting in inability to carry on any physical activity without discomfort. Symptoms of cardiac insufficiency or of the anginal syndrome may be present even at rest. If any physical activity is undertaken, discomfort is increased.	Inability to carry on any physical activity without discomfort; anginal syndrome may be present at rest.	Patients cannot or do not perform to completion activities requiring >2 metabolic equivalents. Cannot carry out activities listed above (specific activity scale III).	Patients with advanced structural heart disease and marked symptoms of HF at rest despite maximal medical therapy and who require specialized interventions.	Extreme limitation; dependent; almost housebound.	NYHA FC IV symptoms Severe aortic enlargement Arrhythmias refractory to treatment Severe hypoxemia (almost always associated with cyanosis) Severe pulmonary hypertension Eisenmenger syndrome Refractory end-organ dysfunction

Abbreviations: AP, anatomic and physiologic; HF, heart failure; NYHA, New York Heart Association.

with age: from around 1% for those aged less than 55 years to greater than 10% in those aged 70 years or over.[7] Therefore, HF is primarily considered to be a disease affecting the elderly, and most HF studies are focused on this group. However, several reports suggest that the incidence of HF among the elderly is decreasing, whereas an increasing number of younger persons develop the condition.[20,21] This shift in the age at onset is mostly related to increasing numbers of patients with ischemic heart disease but also to patients with CHD.[21] Compared with acquired heart disease, the occurrence of HF in ACHD patients is much less, although it is rapidly increasing both in quantity and complexity.

Using administrative health databases, the incidence of HF hospitalization was estimated between 1.2 and 3.16‰ person-year (**Table 2**).[22–24] Although it could offer some indication of the approximate incidence of the condition, this type of data is influenced by the reality that not all patients with HF are hospitalized and not all HF episodes require treatment as inpatients. Compared with age-matched controls, patients with ACHD have a much higher risk of HF. In the Swedish registry, the highest risk of developing HF was found in patients with complex CHD lesions and was strongly age-dependent, with the highest risk found in the youngest age groups. One in fifteen patients with CHD were at risk of developing HF before the age of 42 years, a risk that was 105.7 times higher compared with controls.[3] The prevalence of HF progressively rises with advancing age, with 35% of HF cases being reported in individuals aged more than 65 years.[25,26] Complex CHD is particularly prone to HF events, especially in subgroups of patients with transposition of the great arteries, Fontan circulation, tetralogy of Fallot (one of the largest HF groups in ACHD), atrioventricular septal defect, and cyanotic CHD.[25,26]

End-stage HF is rapidly becoming the leading cause of mortality in the vulnerable ACHD population.[4] According to retrospective data from the Mayo Clinic, the estimated annual incidence of advanced HF in ACHD is 1.1%. This rate was notably higher among patients with a systemic right ventricle (10-year cumulative incidence of 18%) and Fontan palliation/unrepaired single ventricle (10-year cumulative incidence of 24%).[18] These rates significantly exceed those reported in the community, even among elderly patients aged more than 80 years.[32]

Important insights into the prevalence of HF are provided by studies investigating the causes of mortality in ACHD. Usually, only the primary or immediate cause of death is recorded, potentially leading to an underestimation of the true mortality related to HF. Raissadati and colleagues used an extensive nationwide Finnish data set, including 10,964 patients who survived the initial corrective procedure for CHD and were followed up to 45 years post-operation. The results showed that 43% of the late deaths in patients with a CHD were associated with HF. It is worth noting that this figure may not accurately reflect the mortality associated with HF in ACHD, as some patients who died suddenly due to cardiac arrest or perioperative events may have had HF as an additional underlying condition.[33]

Similarly, Oechslin and colleagues conducted a study on 2609 ACHD patients, revealing that 199 of them died at an average age of 37 years, with HF being the cause of death in 21% of cases.[34] Patients with atrioventricular septal defect and complete transposition of the great arteries experienced HF as the primary cause of death. According to a study based on the Dutch CONgenital CORvitia registry, chronic HF was responsible for 26% of deaths in ACHD patients, with an average age of 51 years. Historical factors such as arrhythmias, endocarditis, myocardial infarction, systemic hypertension, and pulmonary hypertension were identified as significant predictors for mortality associated with HF. This condition was prominently seen in cases of univentricular hearts, systemic right ventricles, tetralogy of Fallot, and atrioventricular septal defect.[35] Study based on the German National Registry for CHD confirmed previous observations and provided temporal perspectives on HF-related mortality within ACHD. Between 2001 and 2015, HF-associated mortality increased from 23% to 30%. This increase could potentially be attributed to an aging population with increasing disease complexity. Eisenmenger syndrome, univentricular hearts, systemic right ventricles, and Ebstein's anomaly were significantly associated with mortality.[5] The study conducted at the Royal Brompton Hospital monitored 6969 adults (average age 30 years) from 1991 to 2013. As anticipated, the primary causes of mortality included chronic HF (42%), sudden cardiac death, and mortality from extracardiac factors. Nevertheless, perioperative mortality linked with ACHD was relatively low, albeit with possible referral bias. The study also noticed a significant increase in HF-related deaths as patients living with CHD aged, particularly in cases of complex CHD.[4]

Mortality data are conceptually related to advances in medical care. Mortality in HF remains high and in recent years has been ≈50% at 5 years.[36] These results are even worse in ACHD-related HF, with all-cause mortality after a first HF admission reaching 117 deaths per 100

Table 2
Selected studies reporting on the incidence, prevalence, and mortality of heart failure–related adult congenital heart disease

Diagnostic Criteria	Author, Publication Year	Years Studied	Incidence (‰ Person-Years)	Prevalence	Population Source	Mortality
Non-standardized Criteria						
ICD codes	Zomer et al,[24] 2013	1995–2007	1.2		Dutch CONCOR registry	24% within 1 y and 35% within 3 y after HF admission
ICD codes	Rodriguez et al,[27] 2013	2007		20% of ACHD hospitalization	National Inpatient Sample hospitalization rate	4.1% of HFH (OR 3.3, 95% CI 2.6–4.1, compared with ACHD without HF)
ICD codes	Burchill et al,[25] 2018	1998–2011		91% increase in HFH	National Inpatient Sample hospitalization rate[a]	
ICD codes	Agarwal et al,[28] 2019	2005–2012			California State Inpatient database (excluding ASD)	3% during first HFH, 6.8% during readmission
ICD codes	Burstein et al,[29] 2020	2006–2016		46% increase in HFH after ED visits	Nationwide Emergency Department Sample and Nationwide Inpatient Sample[a]	4.8% of ACHD-HF patients after emergency department visits
ICD codes	Cohen et al,[22] 2020	1995–2010	1.81		Quebec CHD database	
ICD codes	Bergh et al,[23] 2023	1970–2017	3.16	7.8%	Swedish National Patient Register and Cause of Death Register	
ICD codes	Tsang et al,[30] 2021	1994–2018			Ontario Health Insurance	117 per 1000 person-years

Standardized criteria					
Acute HF according to ESC guidelines	Moussa et al,[31] 2017	2013–2015	11.6%	Hospitalizations records at Hôpital Européen Georges Pompidou	20% at 18 months
ACHD working group and HF association of ESC criteria	Arnaert et al,[26] 2021	2001–2019	6.4%	Hospitalizations records at University Hospitals Leuven	40.6 per 1000 patient years

Abbreviations: ASD, atrial septal defect; CHD, congenital heart defect; CONCOR, CONgenital CORvitia; ED, emergency department; ESC, European Society of Cardiology; HFH, heart failure hospitalization; ICD, International Classification of Disease.

[a] Atrial septal defect, bicuspid aortic valve, aortic stenosis, and unspecified congenital anomalies were excluded.

person-years (or 58.5% at 5 years).[30] The onset of HF in ACHD increases the risk of death by two to four times compared with ACHD patients without HF[26–28,30,37] and progression to advanced HF is associated with a sixfold increase in the risk of death.[18] These findings are sobering and underscore that despite advances in management, survival after diagnosis of HF remains poor. Mortality is indeed highest at 30 days, which includes in-hospital mortality. After that, it rapidly declines and tends to plateau at around 10 years following HF episodes (**Fig. 2**A).[28–30,37] However, when comparing mortality in HF patients with and without ACHD, the graphical representation of time-dependent-adjusted hazard ratios exhibits a U-shaped trend (**Fig. 2**B). This indicates a subsequent rise of mortality related to HF in elderly patients with CHD.[30] This trend mainly affects patients with intermediate and high-complexity ACHD and was obtained after adjusting for patient-level and center-level factors.[29,30]

HOSPITALIZATIONS AND HEALTH RESOURCES USE

To understand hospitalization data accurately, it is necessary to explore the terminology concisely. Within the literature, data presentations may be based on the first hospitalization related to HF, which can serve as a proxy for incidence date. Readmissions may be related to HF or caused by other factors. It is essential to distinguish between hospitalizations of HF patients and those which are directly caused by HF. This distinction is significant as HF patients often suffer from multiple comorbidities, which can result in hospitalization for conditions other than HF. In addition, it can be challenging to pinpoint the exact reason for hospitalization due to various factors, including coding practices that prioritize reimbursement and other clinical motives that often coexist among fragile HF patients.

Not surprisingly, HF is increasingly recognized as a major health care issue in ACHD patients. Analysis of the Nationwide Inpatient Sample revealed a notable increase in hospitalizations for ACHD-related HF, with a remarkable 91% escalation in annual cases from 1998 to 2011. In contrast, hospitalizations for non-ACHD HF experienced a comparatively modest increase of 21% over the same period (**Fig. 3**).[25]

HF accounted for almost 20% to 30% of ACHD hospitalizations.[25,27] Patients with ACHD and HF consume more health care resources than those with non-ACHD HF. They are admitted more frequently to the emergency department, their hospitalizations result in longer hospital stays and increased hospital costs. One-quarter of ACHD-HF cases require intensive care, and they are more likely to undergo noninvasive and invasive hemodynamic testing, electrical cardioversion, coronary, and valvular intervention and receive cardiac resynchronization/defibrillator devices and mechanical circulatory support.[25,28–31] Although the number of hospitalizations due to ACHD-HF may increase at a faster rate compared with non-ACHD HF over time, the proportion of ACHD-HF cases receiving a ventricular assist device or transplant has decreased.[29]

The estimated 30-day readmission rate for HF in ACHD was 22.7%, which was lower than non-ACHD patients even after adjustment.[28] Nevertheless, the study by Tsang and colleagues examined the readmissions of ACHD patients due to HF with those of HF patients without ACHD. The analysis was carried out after matching these two groups based on age, sex, and the year of their first hospitalization for HF. ACHD patients with HF were more likely to be readmitted with HF than patients with HF but without ACHD within 30 days of their first HF hospitalization, with a persistent trend continuing up to the 20-year follow-up period.[30] In Zomer and colleagues study the cumulative

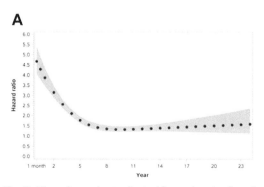
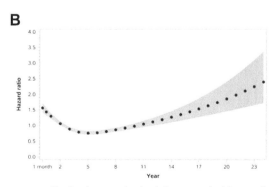

Fig. 2. Time-dependent-adjusted hazard ratios for all-cause mortality in the matched adult congenital heart disease (ACHD) cohort with and without heart failure (HF) (*A*), and in matched HF cohort with and without ACHD (*B*) based on Tsang and colleagues.[30]

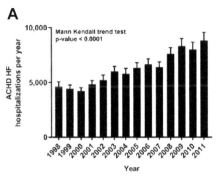
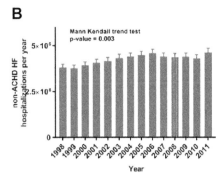

Fig. 3. Adult congenital heart disease (ACHD; *A*) versus non-ACHD (*B*) heart failure (HF) annual hospitalization trends, 1998 to 2011.[25]

risk of readmission for HF was 23% after 1 year,[24] and this risk may rise with the age of the patient. According to Wang and colleagues, who analyzed the Quebec CHD database of patients who experienced their first-ever hospitalization for HF at an age greater than 40, the risk of readmission within 1 year was found to be 48.8%.[38] Moreover, repeat hospitalizations due to HF within the past 12 months were linked to increased mortality risk.[37] It is noteworthy that the risk of readmission during the second week was at its peak, decreased by 50% by the eighth week, followed by stabilization from the twenty-seventh week onward. The investigation recognized three distinct timeframes: the initial attentiveness stage (weeks 1–8), a transitional phase (weeks 9–27), and a stable phase (weeks 28–52). Reductions in readmission risks were related to a history of medical interventions within the past year. It was observed that during the initial observation phase, longer duration of hospital stays were associated with reduced readmission risks.[38]

These findings underscore the substantial burden of HF in ACHD and the critical need for dedicated resources and multidisciplinary interventions, facilitated by adult CHD-HF clinic teams[39,40]

CAUSES OF HEART FAILURE, RISK FACTORS, PREDICTION, AND PREVENTION
Causes of Heart Failure and Risk Factors

Identifying risk factors for adverse outcomes and developing predictive models would allow early identification of high-risk patients and targeted interventions. Moreover, the concept of attributable risk provides a clear understanding of the direct effects of the exposure by emphasizing the additional risk of disease among the exposed group compared with the unexposed group. In ACHD, the causes of HF are variable and closely related to the underlying pathophysiology of the heart. In

the study by Zomer and colleagues, risk factors for HF admission were a diagnosis of univentricular heart, transposition of the great arteries, atrioventricular septal defect, and tetralogy of Fallot. In addition to the underlying cardiac diagnosis, the presence of multiple defects, previous surgery, and pacemaker implantation in childhood were associated with a higher risk of HF.[24] A systematic review has summarized risk factors for HF in ACHD patients.[41] Although a wide variation in population characteristics, follow-up, outcome of interest, and candidate risk factors was observed between studies, certain variables were more frequently considered as predictors of HF. They were age, sex (male), CHD lesion characteristics, NYHA functional class and systemic ventricle function.[41] It is worth noting that traditional risk factors, such as hypertension and diabetes mellitus, are not uncommon in patients with ACHD HF. They coexist with CHD and can interact with one another to increase the likelihood of developing HF.[22,25] The same consideration applies to multimorbidity which is quite prevalent in ACHD with HF. Cardiac arrhythmias were found to play a notable role in the genesis of HF in ACHD[42] as well as pulmonary arterial hypertension, coronary artery disease, liver disease, and chronic kidney disease.[22,25,31] These observations deserve further investigations.

Risk Models and Predictive Equations

Two studies developed a prediction model in patients with ACHD[22,43,44] and two other studies applied HF models developed in the general population.[13,45] Baggen and colleagues and Geenen and colleagues developed the prediction models to predict the 4-year and 1-year risk probability of death, HF, or arrhythmia from a single center database. The final models included age, CHD (only in the 4-year prediction models of outcomes), NYHA class, medication use, reinterventions, body mass index, and BNP (in the 4- and 1-year prediction model of outcomes). The models showed a good performance in predicting HF and had been externally validated.[43,44] The second model was developed from the Quebec CHD databases and predicted the 1 year of incident HF hospitalization. It included age $\geq$ 50 years, male sex, CHD lesion severity, recent 12-month HF hospitalization, pulmonary arterial hypertension, chronic kidney disease, coronary artery disease, systemic arterial hypertension, and diabetes mellitus. A risk score system based on adjusted odds ratios was created and showed an excellent prediction performance. However, the model has not yet undergone external validation.

Lin and colleagues[45] and Stefanescu and colleagues[13] presented the performance of the Heart Failure Survival Score (HFSS) and the SHFM, respectively, in a cohort of patients with ACHD. Both studies used composite outcome including death, cardiac transplant, ventricular assist device placement, arrhythmia requiring treatment, and cardiovascular admissions. The HFSS did not adequately risk stratify ACHD, whose heterogeneous pathophysiology differs from that of the acquired HF population. The SHFM discriminated individuals with CHD at risk of adverse outcomes including HF and poor cardiopulmonary performance. However, it did not allow for the specific identification of the risk for HF alone.

Perspectives

This review does not cover an extensive analysis of emerging risk factors of HF in ACHD because there are limited epidemiologic data on this topic concerning HF in ACHD. This is highlighted to emphasize the necessity for additional research in these areas. The lack of data on racial disparities in HF outcomes in ACHD is a significant gap in our understanding of this complex disease. Recent research has highlighted the growing concern about disparities in HF[46] and CHD[47–49] care and outcomes for racial/ethnic minorities. This lack of data is a critical issue that needs to be addressed in future research efforts. Understanding how racial and ethnic factors may affect the prevalence, progression, and management of HF in patients with ACHD is critical to providing equitable health care and improving patient outcomes. This research will play an important role in advancing the field and ensuring that health care is more inclusive and equitable for all.

Several emerging risk factors have been explored in small population and included fibrosis,[50] biological biomarkers,[51] and more recently multiomics.[52] The contribution of genetic factors in HF of patients with transposition of the great arteries has recently been investigated. A genome-wide significant locus on chromosome 10 and 18 suggestive loci has been identified for association with the combined endpoint of HF, ventricular arrhythmias, and mortality. The addition of genetic information significantly improved risk prediction compared with the use of clinical risk factors alone.[52] The next step in risk assessment for ACHD patients may be the integrated approach of multidimensional data.

SUMMARY

Based on the available information, HF seems to be prevalent in people with ACHD, with a lifetime incidence of at least 30% in those with complex CHD. HF is one of the leading causes of death in this group and its prevalence is increasing as patients age. As more people with complex heart disease live longer and the ACHD population in general increases, the potential for an outbreak of HF in this population is a looming concern. To gain a full understanding, continued efforts are needed to accurately assess the incidence and prevalence of HF in different age groups and across the spectrum of ACHD. It is worth noting that existing data may not fully capture the current needs of ACHD patients, particularly in the modern era of improved ACHD management and surgical expertise. Furthermore, the advent of interventional techniques may facilitate early hemodynamic correction, thereby avoiding some of the documented long-term complications, including HF. Therefore, collaborative initiatives to collect contemporary data on the incidence and prevalence of HF in patients with ACHD are imperative. Improving the identification of high-risk patients, early detection practices, and anticipation of novel therapeutic opportunities are urgent imperatives to prevent a severe escalation of HF-related morbidity and mortality in this specific population.

CLINICS CARE POINTS

- Comprehensive ACHD-HF recognition: Recognize the multifactorial nature of heart failure (HF) in adults with congenital heart disease (ACHD). Consider diverse anatomic substrates and pathophysiology, and use a comprehensive clinical diagnosis integrating epidemiological definitions, HF presentations, stages, and cardiac assessments. Variability in definitions may lead to underreporting.

- Highlight the significance of clinical diagnosis in ACHD-HF. Avoid sole reliance on a single

test, consider age-related symptom variations, and utilize the NYHA classification as
a valuable tool correlating with exercise measures and long-term mortality.

- Acknowledge burden and advocate for resources in ACHD-HF: Acknowledge the substantial HF burden in ACHD. Emphasize the
need for dedicated resources and multidisciplinary interventions. Establish ACHD-HF
clinic teams to address specific healthcare
needs and resource patterns.

- Recognize predictive model limitations in
ACHD-HF: Recognize limitations in existing
predictive models for stratifying HF risk in
ACHD. Consider the unique pathophysiology
and explore the need for refined models
tailored to this population.

DISCLOSURE

The authors have no conflict of interest to declare.

REFERENCES

1. Marelli AJ, Ionescu-Ittu R, Mackie AS, et al. Lifetime
prevalence of congenital heart disease in the general population from 2000 to 2010. Circulation
2014;130(9):749–56.
2. Egbe AC, Miranda WR, Jain CC, et al. Temporal
Changes in Clinical Characteristics and Outcomes
of Adults With Congenital Heart Disease. Am Heart
J 2023;264:1–9.
3. Gilljam T, Mandalenakis Z, Dellborg M, et al. Development of heart failure in young patients with
congenital heart disease: a nation-wide cohort
study. Open Heart 2019;6(1):e000858.
4. Diller GP, Kempny A, Alonso-Gonzalez R, et al. Survival Prospects and Circumstances of Death in
Contemporary Adult Congenital Heart Disease Patients Under Follow-Up at a Large Tertiary Centre.
Circulation 2015;132(22):2118–25.
5. Engelings CC, Helm PC, Abdul-Khaliq H, et al.
Cause of death in adults with congenital heart disease - An analysis of the German National Register
for Congenital Heart Defects. Int J Cardiol 2016;
211:31–6.
6. Poole Wilson PA, Buller NP. Causes of symptoms in
chronic congestive heart failure and implications for
treatment. Am J Cardiol 1988;62(2):31A–4A.
7. McDonagh TA, Metra M, Adamo M, et al. ESC
Guidelines for the diagnosis and treatment of acute
and chronic heart failure. Eur Heart J 2021;42(36):
3599–726.
8. Hunt SA, Baker DW, Chin MH, et al. ACC/AHA
Guidelines for the Evaluation and Management of
Chronic Heart Failure in the Adult: Executive

Summary A Report of the American College of
Cardiology/American Heart Association Task Force
on Practice Guidelines (Committee to Revise the
1995 Guidelines for the Evaluation and Management of Heart Failure): Developed in Collaboration
With the International Society for Heart and Lung
Transplantation; Endorsed by the Heart Failure Society of America. Circulation 2001;104(24):
2996–3007.
9. Budts W, Roos-Hesselink J, Rädle-Hurst T, et al.
Treatment of heart failure in adult congenital heart
disease: a position paper of the Working Group of
Grown-Up Congenital Heart Disease and the Heart
Failure Association of the European Society of Cardiology. Eur Heart J 2016;37(18):1419–27.
10. Gratz A, Hess J, Hager A. Self-estimated physical
functioning poorly predicts actual exercise capacity
in adolescents and adults with congenital heart disease. Eur Heart J 2009;30(4):497–504.
11. Bredy C, Ministeri M, Kempny A, et al. New York
Heart Association (NYHA) classification in adults
with congenital heart disease: relation to objective
measures of exercise and outcome. Eur Heart J
Qual Care Clin Outcomes 2018;4(1):51–8.
12. Lachtrupp CL, Valente AM, Gurvitz M, et al. Associations Between Clinical Outcomes and a Recently
Proposed Adult Congenital Heart Disease Anatomic
and Physiological Classification System. J Am Heart
Assoc 2021;10(18):e021345.
13. Stefanescu A, Macklin EA, Lin E, et al. Usefulness of
the Seattle Heart Failure Model to identify adults with
congenital heart disease at high risk of poor
outcome. Am J Cardiol 2014;113(5):865–70.
14. Stout KK, Daniels CJ, Aboulhosn JA, et al. 2018
AHA/ACC Guideline for the Management of Adults
With Congenital Heart Disease: A Report of the
American College of Cardiology/American Heart Association Task Force on Clinical Practice Guidelines.
Circulation 2019;139(14):e698–800.
15. Stout KK, Broberg CS, Book WM, et al. Chronic
Heart Failure in Congenital Heart Disease: A Scientific Statement From the American Heart Association. Circulation 2016;133(8):770–801.
16. Nomenclature and Criteria for Diagnosis of Diseases of the Heart. J Am Med Assoc 1940;
114(20):2054.
17. Alsaied T, Rathod RH, Aboulhosn JA, et al. Reaching
consensus for unified medical language in Fontan
care. ESC Heart Fail 2021;8(5):3894–905.
18. Egbe AC, Miranda WR, Jain CC, et al. Incidence
and Outcomes of Advanced Heart Failure in Adults
With Congenital Heart Disease. Circ Heart Fail
2022;15(12):e009675.
19. Tsao CW, Aday AW, Almarzooq ZI, et al. Heart Disease and Stroke Statistics-2023 Update: A Report
From the American Heart Association. Circulation
2023;147(8):e93–621.

20. Christiansen MN, Køber L, Weeke P, et al. Age-Specific Trends in Incidence, Mortality, and Comorbidities of Heart Failure in Denmark, 1995 to 2012. Circulation 2017;135(13):1214–23.

21. Lecoeur E, Domengé O, Fayol A, et al. Epidemiology of heart failure in young adults: a French nationwide cohort study. Eur Heart J 2022;44(5):383–92.

22. Cohen S, Liu A, Wang F, et al. Risk prediction models for heart failure admissions in adults with congenital heart disease. Int J Cardiol 2021;322:149–57.

23. Bergh N, Skoglund K, Fedchenko M, et al. Risk of Heart Failure in Congenital Heart Disease: A Nationwide Register-Based Cohort Study. Circulation 2023; 147(12):982–4.

24. Zomer AC, Vaartjes I, van der Velde ET, et al. Heart failure admissions in adults with congenital heart disease; risk factors and prognosis. Int J Cardiol 2013;168(3):2487–93.

25. Burchill LJ, Gao L, Kovacs AH, et al. Hospitalization Trends and Health Resource Use for Adult Congenital Heart Disease-Related Heart Failure. J Am Heart Assoc 2018;7(15):e008775.

26. Arnaert S, De Meester P, Troost E, et al. Heart failure related to adult congenital heart disease: prevalence, outcome and risk factors. ESC Heart Fail 2021;8(4):2940–50.

27. Rodriguez FH, Moodie DS, Parekh DR, et al. Outcomes of heart failure-related hospitalization in adults with congenital heart disease in the United States. Congenit Heart Dis 2013;8(6):513–9.

28. Agarwal A, Dudley CW, Nah G, et al. Clinical Outcomes During Admissions for Heart Failure Among Adults With Congenital Heart Disease. J Am Heart Assoc 2019;8(16):e012595.

29. Burstein DS, Rossano JW, Griffis H, et al. Greater admissions, mortality and cost of heart failure in adults with congenital heart disease. Heart 2021; 107(10):807–13.

30. Tsang W, Silversides CK, Rashid M, et al. Outcomes and healthcare resource utilization in adult congenital heart disease patients with heart failure. ESC Heart Fail 2021;8(5):4139–51.

31. Moussa NB, Karsenty C, Pontnau F, et al. Characteristics and outcomes of heart failure-related hospitalization in adults with congenital heart disease. Arch Cardiovasc Dis 2017;110(5):283–91.

32. Dunlay SM, Roger VL, Killian JM, et al. Advanced Heart Failure Epidemiology and Outcomes: A Population-Based Study. JACC Heart Fail 2021; 9(10):722–32.

33. Raissadati A, Nieminen H, Haukka J, et al. Late Causes of Death After Pediatric Cardiac Surgery: A 60-Year Population-Based Study. J Am Coll Cardiol 2016;68(5):487–98.

34. Oechslin EN, Harrison DA, Connelly MS, et al. Mode of death in adults with congenital heart disease. Am J Cardiol 2000;86(10):1111–6.

35. Verheugt CL, Uiterwaal CSPM, van der Velde ET, et al. Mortality in adult congenital heart disease. Eur Heart J 2010;31(10):1220–9.

36. Roger VL. Epidemiology of Heart Failure: A Contemporary Perspective. Circ Res 2021;128(10): 1421–34.

37. Wang F, Liu A, Brophy JM, et al. Determinants of Survival in Older Adults With Congenital Heart Disease Newly Hospitalized for Heart Failure. Circ Heart Fail 2020;13(8):e006490.

38. Wang F, Sterling LH, Liu A, et al. Risk of readmission after heart failure hospitalization in older adults with congenital heart disease. Int J Cardiol 2020;320: 70–6.

39. Ladouceur M. Heart failure in adults with congenital heart disease: a call for action. Heart 2021;107(10): 774–5.

40. Crossland DS, Van De Bruaene A, Silversides CK, et al. Heart Failure in Adult Congenital Heart Disease: From Advanced Therapies to End-of-Life Care. Can J Cardiol 2019;35(12):1723–39.

41. Wang F, Harel-Sterling L, Cohen S, et al. Heart failure risk predictions in adult patients with congenital heart disease: a systematic review. Heart 2019; 105(21):1661–9.

42. Moore JP, Marelli A, Burchill LJ, et al. Management of Heart Failure With Arrhythmia in Adults With Congenital Heart Disease: JACC State-of-the-Art Review. J Am Coll Cardiol 2022;80(23):2224–38.

43. Baggen VJM, Venema E, Živná R, et al. Development and validation of a risk prediction model in patients with adult congenital heart disease. Int J Cardiol 2019;276:87–92.

44. Geenen LW, Opotowsky AR, Lachtrupp C, et al. Tuning and external validation of an adult congenital heart disease risk prediction model. Eur Heart J Qual Care Clin Outcomes 2022;8(1):70–8.

45. Lin EY, Cohen HW, Bhatt AB, et al. Predicting Outcomes Using the Heart Failure Survival Score in Adults with Moderate or Complex Congenital Heart Disease. Congenit Heart Dis 2015;10(5):387–95.

46. Piña IL, Jimenez S, Lewis EF, et al. Race and Ethnicity in Heart Failure: JACC Focus Seminar 8/ 9. J Am Coll Cardiol 2021;78(25):2589–98.

47. Bhamidipati CM, Garcia IC, Kim B, et al. Racial Disparity: The Adult Congenital Heart Disease Surgery Perspective. Pediatr Cardiol 2022. https://doi. org/10.1007/s00246-022-03087-5.

48. Lopez KN, Morris SA, Sexson Tejtel SK, et al. US Mortality Attributable to Congenital Heart Disease Across the Lifespan From 1999 Through 2017 Exposes Persistent Racial/Ethnic Disparities. Circulation 2020;142(12):1132–47.

49. Jackson JL, Morack J, Harris M, et al. Racial disparities in clinic follow-up early in life among survivors of congenital heart disease. Congenit Heart Dis 2019; 14(2):305–10.

50. Gordon B, González-Fernández V, Dos-Subirà L. Myocardial fibrosis in congenital heart disease. Front Pediatr 2022;10:965204.

51. Baggen VJM, van den Bosch AE, Eindhoven JA, et al. Prognostic Value of N-Terminal Pro-B-Type Natriuretic Peptide, Troponin-T, and Growth-Differentiation Factor 15 in Adult Congenital Heart Disease. Circulation 2017; 135(3):264–79.

52. Woudstra OI, Skoric-Milosavljevic D, Mulder BJM, et al. Common genetic variants improve risk stratification after the atrial switch operation for transposition of the great arteries. Int J Cardiol 2023;371:153–9.

The Pathophysiology(ies) of Heart Failure in Adults with Congenital Heart Disease

Alexander R. Opotowsky, MD, MMSc

KEYWORDS

- Heart failure • Congenital heart disease • Adult congenital heart disease • Pathophysiology
- Pulmonary vascular disease • Right heart failure • Valve disease

KEY POINTS

- Adults with congenital heart disease (CHD) exhibit a range of heart failure pathophysiologies, often complicating straightforward application of existing heart failure definitions and guideline-directed management.
- A subset of patients experienced heart failure for reasons similar to acquired forms of heart failure in adults, such as ventricular dysfunction and valve disease.
- Other causes of heart failure, however, are also commonly present such as venous insufficiency and lymphatic dysfunction.
- The chronicity of CHD and the long-term cumulative impact of subclinical hemodynamic abnormalities are associated with end-organ effects that may mimic heart failure or exacerbate its expression.

INTRODUCTION

With improved medical and surgical care, most individuals born with congenital heart disease (CHD) now live well into adulthood. As this heterogeneous population has aged, there has been a concomitant increase in the incidence and prevalence of heart failure. Taken as a whole, heart failure is the most common cause of death among adults with CHD. This statement, however, obscures how difficult it is in the context of CHD to define exactly what we mean by heart failure. Heart failure is a clinical syndrome and may result from a wide array of causes, with variable pathophysiology requiring distinct management and diverse manifestations. Other diagnoses which often occur in the context of CHD may present similarly to heart failure and these same diagnoses also often play a role in causing or exacerbating the presentation of heart failure.

This article describes proposed definitions of heart failure as they relate to consideration of pathophysiology, the range of hemodynamic pathophysiologic mechanisms that underlie heart failure, common heart failure mimics, and examples of scenarios often associated with heart failure in adults with CHD.

DEFINITIONS AND PATHOPHYSIOLOGY

Heart failure is characterized by typical symptoms (eg, dyspnea, fatigue) and signs (eg, dependent edema, crackles) of congestion or low cardiac output, resulting from a cardiac disorder, whether structural or functional. Recent professional society statements and guidelines, however, have been more proactive in identifying individuals with heart failure to facilitate prevention. Heart failure has been classified by stages, with stage A and stage B describing individuals who do not, in fact, have the clinical syndrome of heart failure.[1] Stage

Cincinnati Adult Congenital Heart Disease Program, Department of Pediatrics, Heart Institute, Cincinnati Children's Hospital, University of Cincinnati College of Medicine, 3333 Burnet Avenue, MLC 2003, Cincinnati, OH 45229, USA
E-mail address: sasha.opotowsky@cchmc.org

Heart Failure Clin 20 (2024) 129–136
https://doi.org/10.1016/j.hfc.2024.01.001
1551-7136/24/© 2024 Elsevier Inc. All rights reserved.

A refers to those "at risk for heart failure" without symptoms or apparent structural abnormalities who are at risk for heart failure (eg, diabetes mellitus or obesity). Stage B describes "pre-heart failure" individuals who do not have current or prior symptoms of heart failure but who do have structural heart disease, elevated filling pressures or other risk factors. Stages C describes patients with "current or prior symptoms and/or signs of heart failure", while stage D indicates those with severe manifestations of heart failure despite medical therapy.

As described in published reviews and statements, this classification does not neatly fit for CHD.[2,3] Since CHD is defined by the presence of structural heart disease at birth, all have at least stage B heart failure. Presumably, those with heart failure during infancy who were subsequently repaired (eg, ventricular septal defect [VSD]) would be classified as stage C heart failure. Inconsistent with this, however, a proposed 'universal' definition of heart failure described these stages but also made a specific note about CHD, specifying that only "some types of CHD can result in heart failure."[1] This latter perspective is more intuitive, since it is difficult to see how a young man with a VSD repaired in infancy for failure-to-thrive should be considered to have heart failure at all in the context of excellent functional capacity, reassuring current cardiac status (eg, normal ventricular function, normal valve function), and an excellent prognosis. As such, caution should be exercised not to apply existing heart failure definitions (or guidelines) literally and without thought to the underlying meaning in the larger context when applied to individuals with CHD.

The care for adults with CHD is informed by knowledge deriving from experiences with and literature on both adult heart failure and pediatric CHD. This leads to tensions, because their conceptual and practical approaches are strikingly different. While the management of adult heart failure focuses on guideline-directed medical therapy, the management of CHD in children, conversely, tends to focus on surgical or transcatheter intervention to address residual structural lesions that may cause or be associated with long-term risk for heart failure and other adverse outcomes.[2] Pivotal trials in adult heart failure have not been replicated in pediatric cohorts, and there is much less evidence that medical therapy provides clinically meaningful benefit, whether to prevent or treat heart failure, for children with or without CHD or adults with CHD.[4–7]

Further, the usual definitions and classifications of heart failure are not conducive to clinical research or other systematic efforts to improve our understanding of heart failure in adults with CHD. Directly applying this heart failure staging system classifies too many otherwise well individuals as having stage C heart failure, as above. Investigators analyzing data on heart failure in CHD have attempted to address this in various ways. One study, for example, defined heart failure in adults with CHD as an N-terminal-pro-brain natriuretic peptide (NT-proBNP) level of 100 pg/mL or more and a peak oxygen consumption (V_{O_2}) of 25 mL/kg/min or lower.[8] Using this definition, the investigators reported an overall heart failure prevalence of 26% (89 of 345 patients) in a group of young adult patients with mostly moderate or severely complex CHD. While this definition would no doubt be associated with the risk of having or developing heart failure, neither NT-proBNP nor peak V_{O_2} nor their combination is sufficient to define the clinical syndrome of heart failure. Only 12 of 89 (14%) patients classified as having heart failure in this study were prescribed a diuretic, which would suggest that many of these patients did not have clinical heart failure. Equally relevant, some patients with clinical heart failure would not be captured by this or any definition described by objectively measured quantitative data. Quantitative measurements without reference to symptoms or signs of clinical heart failure will inevitably imply either spurious or trivial associations. In the example above, those meeting the definition of heart failure were older. That may be true, but even among those who do not have heart failure and do not ever develop heart failure, aging is associated with higher NT-proBNP and lower peak V_{O_2}.

Individuals with CHD may also experience noncardiac clinical deterioration reflecting the cumulative long-term impact of CHD (**Fig. 1**). While these are not rightly considered as 'heart failure,' it is important to consider how chronic, compensated cardiovascular dysfunction (subclinical heart failure) may lead to adverse outcomes in the absence of clinical heart failure. Examples include the development of ascites or hepatocellular carcinoma in those with Fontan circulation or in situ thrombosis and hemoptysis in Eisenmenger syndrome. Each of these phenomena may be traced to long-standing elevations in venous pressure and low or limited cardiac output, as seen with heart failure but also often with additional predisposing factors.

The earlier discussion of shortcomings in defining heart failure in adults with CHD does not imply that prior work was flawed but rather emphasizes the intrinsic challenges and tradeoffs necessary as we define and study heart failure in this distinct and diverse population. The term heart failure, whether throughout this review or in the broader literature, may be used to represent different things in different contexts (eg., with

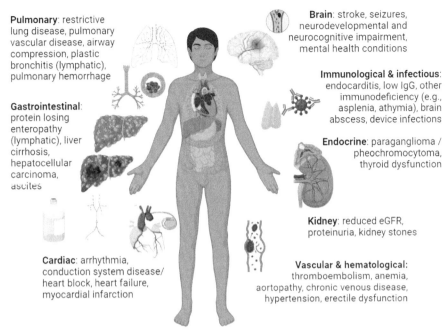

Pulmonary: restrictive lung disease, pulmonary vascular disease, airway compression, plastic bronchitis (lymphatic), pulmonary hemorrhage

Gastrointestinal: protein losing enteropathy (lymphatic), liver cirrhosis, hepatocellular carcinoma, ascites

Cardiac: arrhythmia, conduction system disease/ heart block, heart failure, myocardial infarction

Brain: stroke, seizures, neurodevelopmental and neurocognitive impairment, mental health conditions

Immunological & infectious: endocarditis, low IgG, other immunodeficiency (e.g., asplenia, athymia), brain abscess, device infections

Endocrine: paraganglioma / pheochromocytoma, thyroid dysfunction

Kidney: reduced eGFR, proteinuria, kidney stones

Vascular & hematological: thromboembolism, anemia, aortopathy, chronic venous disease, hypertension, erectile dysfunction

Fig. 1. Long-term sequelae of circulatory dysfunction, but is it heart failure? There exists a broad spectrum of potential long-term consequences of subclinical circulatory and hemodynamic perturbations in this example for individuals with hypoplastic left heart syndrome and an extracardiac Fontan circulation. Because some of these consequences manifest in ways that overlap with heart failure, such as protein-losing enteropathy, cirrhosis, or thyroid dysfunction, it can be challenging to define what comprises heart failure. (Created with BioRender.com.)

different patient groups). As a consequence, care for adults with CHD and heart failure is poorly served by algorithmic decision-making, but rather requires experienced and flexible clinical judgment founded on a deep understanding of underlying pathophysiology.[9]

MECHANISMS OF HEART FAILURE IN ADULTS WITH CONGENITAL HEART DISEASE

Heart failure is, fundamentally, characterized by inadequate cardiac output or elevated venous pressure or both. There is an inconsistent relationship between the degree of hemodynamic impairment and the severity of clinical manifestations; and, a wide array of factors modify the expression of heart failure in an individual. In the following sections selected mechanisms of heart failure among adults with CHD are discussed, focusing on the most common causes as well as those which often have a more prominent role in those with CHD compared with adults acquired forms of heart failure, acknowledging that the probability of these mechanisms is heavily dependent on details of the clinical context (**Table 1**).

a. Systemic ventricular dysfunction
b. Valve stenosis and regurgitation
c. Arrhythmia and conduction system disease

CHD is associated with an increased risk for systemic ventricular dysfunction (systolic and diastolic), valve disease (right-sided or left-sided, stenotic or regurgitant), and arrhythmia (tachyarrhythmia, sinus node dysfunction, and conduction system disease). Any of these can lead to symptoms and signs consistent with heart failure just as they do in acquired heart disease. There is a distinction from acquired heart disease, however, in how much evidence exists to guide indications for invasive intervention or to indicate when "guideline-directed medical therapy" is beneficial in adults with CHD. It does not follow, however, that we should deprive individuals of potentially beneficial therapies because of the absence of robust research in this understudied population. Clinicians must carefully consider whether to extrapolate data on acquired heart failure in the setting of an individual patient's situation, mainly relying on pathophysiology but with further thought given to social, psychological, and financial factors.

For some therapies, extrapolation from extensive experience in acquired adult heart disease to adults with CHD may be straightforward. For example, an implantable hemodynamic monitor should be useful for any individuals in whom the mechanism of heart failure involves elevated pulmonary venous pressure as a central component of the causal

Table 1
Mechanisms of heart failure and similar symptomatology in adults with various forms of congenital heart disease

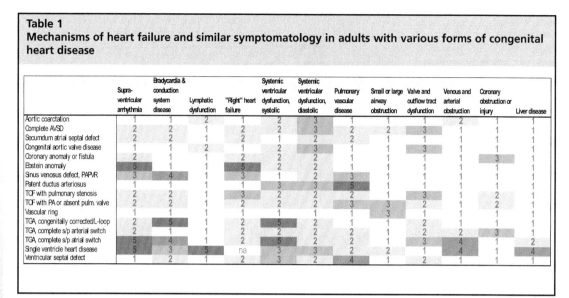

	Supraventricular arrhythmia	Bradycardia & conduction system disease	Lymphatic dysfunction	"Right" heart failure	Systemic ventricular dysfunction, systolic	Systemic ventricular dysfunction, diastolic	Pulmonary vascular disease	Small or large airway obstruction	Valve and outflow tract dysfunction	Venous and arterial obstruction	Coronary obstruction or injury	Liver disease
Aortic coarctation	1	1	1	2	1	2	3	1	1	2	1	1
Complete AVSD	2	2	1	2	2	3	2	2	3	1	1	1
Secundum atrial septal defect	2	2	1	2	1	2	2	1	1	1	1	1
Congenital aortic valve disease	1	1	2	1	2	3	1	1	3	1	1	1
Coronary anomaly or fistula	2	1	1	2	2	2	1	1	1	1	3	1
Ebstein anomaly	5	1	1	5	2	2	1	1	1	1	1	1
Sinus venosus defect, PAPVR	3	4	1	3	1	2	3	1	1	1	1	1
Patent ductus arteriosus	1	1	1	1	3	3	5	1	1	1	1	1
TOF with pulmonary stenosis	2	2	1	3	2	2	2	1	3	1	2	1
TOF with PA or absent pulm. valve	2	2	1	2	2	2	3	3	2	1	2	1
Vascular ring	1	1	1	1	1	1	1	3	1	1	1	1
TGA congenitally corrected/L-loop	2	5	1	2	5	2	1	1	2	1	1	1
TGA complete s/p arterial switch	2	1	1	2	2	2	2	1	2	2	3	1
TGA complete s/p atrial switch	5	4	1	2	5	2	2	1	3	4	1	2
Single ventricle heart disease	5	3	5	na	3	3	2	2	1	4	1	4
Ventricular septal defect	1	2	1	2	3	2	4	1	2	1	1	1

The number in each cell indicates relative risk of heart failure pathophysiology. In some, the risk relates to a shared association (eg, Turner syndrome with aortic valve disease or coarctation). Also, in some cases, risk relates to complications of common interventions.

For most diagnoses, risk also varies by anatomic severity and intervention with exceptions (eg, transposition of the great arteries). For example, tetralogy of Fallot may be associated with varying risk of valve dysfunction and right heart failure depending on underlying anatomy or surgical repair; or a moderate-sized, unrepaired patent ductus arteriosus is associated with high risk of pulmonary vascular disease or heart failure while a silent PDA or a PDA s/p ligation early in life would not. These distinctions are not detailed in this table. Likewise, interpretation and implications vary between diagnoses. For example, the pulmonary vascular disease associated with single-ventricle heart disease is distinct from that associated with shunt lesions, and the numerical severity is not directly comparable.

Abbreviations: AVSD, atrioventricular septal defect; PA, pulmonary atresia; PAPVR, partial anomalous pulmonary venous return; PDA, patent ductus arteriosus; TGA, transposition of the great arteries; TOF, tetralogy of Fallot.

pathway between heart failure and episodic deterioration, and identifying this change early could lead to a proven therapy that could interrupt the decline (eg, dextro-transposition of the great arteries s/p atrial switch with systolic dysfunction). Conversely, the existing data may not directly support how this technology would be helpful for individuals with pulmonary vascular disease (PVD) or the subset of individuals with single ventricular Fontan circulation in whom deterioration is not directly related to elevated pulmonary venous pressure or in whom this relationship may not be amenable to proactive medication titration.

In many cases, though, the causal pathway between intervention and outcome is less intuitive or readily measured. For example, neurohormonal-modifying medications may not be associated with consistently measurable improvement in imaging or biomarkers yet provide substantial long-term benefit in acquired heart failure. There are no consistently dependable surrogate markers of response to the range of heart failure therapies,[10,11] making it impossible to determine whether a specific set of medications provides benefit in an individual with modestly or markedly

distinct pathophysiology, even when the same indications are met.

For example, should every adult with CHD, left ventricular ejection fraction less than 40%, and a history of heart failure symptoms receive guideline-directed medical therapies for heart failure with reduced ejection fraction, including a beta-blocker, angiotensin receptor/neprilysin inhibitor, sodium-glucose cotransporter 2 inhibitor, and aldosterone receptor blocker? Even if symptoms occurred in the distant past, ventricular dysfunction is largely explained by an identifiable structural abnormality (eg, large VSD patch with dyskinesis), and indicators of cardiac function have been stable for many years?

Many reasons caution against dogmatic, unbridled extrapolation. Some of these relate to pathophysiology and pitfalls particular to specific situations. Others relate to differing historical knowledge or time horizons. Acquired heart failure is usually identified because of symptoms, or at least some other reason for investigation. Conversely, ventricular dysfunction in adults with CHD is often identified incidentally as part of standard imaging. The same degree of ventricular dysfunction thus identified may often be associated with strikingly different implications and prognosis, and the benefit of therapies may be overestimated by data from acquired adult heart failure. Further, because of the historical evolution of cardiac surgery, adults with more complex forms of CHD tend to be decades younger, on average, than those with acquired heart failure. Prescribing 4 medications to be taken once or twice every day likely has a greater impact on quality of life and also may be associated with worse adherence overall for younger adults, as has been described in other scenarios such as for antihypertensive medications.[12]

d. Pulmonary vascular disease

Subsets of CHD are associated with an increased risk for PVD, most often related to left-to-right shunting with septal defects, patent ductus arteriosus (PDA), or less common lesions (eg, aortopulmonary window). These shunt lesions are associated with variably increased pulmonary blood flow and pressure, leading to pulmonary vascular remodeling and, consequently, elevated pulmonary resistance. These lesions are associated with different risks for developing PVD, with risk descending from PDA, VSD, sinus venosus defects, and secundum atrial septal defect.

Elevated pulmonary vascular resistance may cause right heart failure, as the right ventricle faces increased afterload. Chronically elevated pulmonary artery pressure also leads to right ventricular hypertrophy and elevated right atrial pressure. In Eisenmenger syndrome, in the context of a patent shunt, the shunt becomes bidirectional or reverses (right-to-left), leading to systemic hypoxemia and cyanosis.[13] As noted earlier, however, the consequences of this extend far beyond these proximate manifestations (see **Fig. 1**).[14]

Other causes of PVD in CHD include segmental pulmonary arterial hypertension, as can happen with tetralogy of Fallot with pulmonary atresia or branch pulmonary artery stenosis.[15] Localized areas of high pressure and abnormal flow lead to microvascular changes consistent with pulmonary arterial hypertension, additive with the increased afterload related to macroscopic pulmonary arterial stenoses.

Beyond the direct effect of increased pulmonary arterial impedance on right ventricular function and, over the long term, structure and adverse ventricular interaction can further constrain the circulation. The right and left ventricles share a common septum and pericardial space. Right ventricular dysfunction can mechanically and hemodynamically affect left ventricular systolic and diastolic function. For example, prolonged right ventricular isovolumic contraction may impinge on early left ventricular filling,[16] mimicking intrinsic left ventricular diastolic dysfunction.

With the Fontan circulation, the absence of a subpulmonary power source (ventricle) means pulmonary blood flow is highly susceptible to any degree of increased impedance, whether due to conduit vessel obstruction or microscopic PVD. The resulting increase in venous pressure and limitation in cardiac output augmentation can increase the risk for other Fontan-related complications (eg, protein-losing enteropathy [PLE], liver congestion), complicating the clinical picture.

e. Arterial or venous pathology

In some forms of CHD, vascular dysfunction and obstruction can have an outsized impact on cardiac output and venous pressure. Arterial obstruction, as in the case of coarctation of the aorta, can cause neurohormonal and other changes leading to systemic hypertension, left ventricular hypertrophy, and left heart failure. In the current era, most patients have had earlier intervention; however, heart failure in early adulthood is now rarely seen with coarctation. Coronary arterial obstruction, whether in the native coronary artery or a conduit (eg, Damus-Kay-Stansel anastomosis), may cause heart failure or similar symptomatology via myocardial ischemia or infarction. Vasodilation and systemic arteriovenous malformations, which may result from liver cirrhosis in the setting of chronic congestion, can be associated with high-output heart failure or, in the context of limited cardiac output, a steal-like phenomenon with normal cardiac output but reduced effective perfusion.

Venous pathophysiology is more often overlooked and misunderstood, both with CHD and in general.[17] It stands to reason that the heart cannot augment cardiac output beyond the amount of blood supplied by the venous return. The low-pressure, high-compliance venous system is susceptible to obstruction. Clinically, this is most common (and most often overlooked) in the context of Fontan circulation (at any point in the pathway, from systemic great veins through pulmonary arteries) and complete transposition of the great arteries after an atrial switch operation.[18,19] Pulmonary venous obstruction is also not infrequent in some forms of CHD and can cause effort intolerance and other symptomatology indistinguishable from heart failure.

f. Lymphatic dysfunction

The lymphatic system is central to maintaining fluid balance and tissue homeostasis, serving to remove excess fluid driven by osmotic and oncotic pressure gradients into the interstitium. In the context of heart failure, relative lymphatic insufficiency can lead to an inability to adequately manage this excess fluid, exacerbating symptoms of volume overload. In the context of heart failure, intact lymphatic function provides a buffer against the development of edema, a cardinal feature of decompensated heart failure.[20,21] Presumably, similar relationships apply to most adults with CHD, though some subgroups also have a genetic predisposition to lymphatic dysfunction that may present with some overlap with the presentation of heart failure (eg, lymphedema with Turner syndrome),[22] while others may experience lymphatic dysfunction due to iatrogenic injury. There are also distinct clinical syndromes in complex CHD related to lymphatic dysfunction that share substantial phenotypic overlap with heart failure, most notably in those with Fontan circulation, The Fontan procedure, performed in children with single-ventricle physiology, is especially prone to PLE and plastic bronchitis, both of which are indicative of severe lymphatic dysfunction. PLE results in significant protein loss via the gastrointestinal tract leading to hypoalbuminemia, edema, and other manifestations (eg, immunodeficiency). While elevated venous pressure may be part of the causal pathway for PLE, there is also thought to be a propensity based on lymphatic development and pathophysiology independent of any contribution of heart failure. Some treatments overlap with those used for heart failure (eg, diuretics, cardiac transplant) while others target entirely unrelated mechanisms (eg, budesonide). Further, there is ongoing investigation of the use of lymphatic interventions to ameliorate the severity of PLE and plastic bronchitis.[23]

While there is increasing appreciation of the role of the lymphatic system in the manifestation of heart failure and related syndromes among adults with CHD, our understanding of lymphatic dysfunction remains far from complete.

g. Iatrogenic

Interventions intended to provide benefit can exacerbate heart failure or can present clinical presentations similar to heart failure. Copious volume resuscitation and mechanical ventilation are common in the setting of surgeries and other procedures. Iatrogenic heart block, sinus node dysfunction, baffle leaks, baffle or vessel obstruction, and other surgical complications can often cause effort intolerance and other symptoms of heart failure. Medications can also cause symptoms of heart failure by diverse mechanisms. For example, beta-blockers may cause dyspnea, sexual dysfunction, and fatigue while dihydropyridine calcium channel blockers or thiazolidinediones may cause edema.

h. Other causes and mimics

Many other diagnoses present with symptoms and signs that overlap with heart failure (**Table 2**). Some of these are more common among those with CHD and some are also associated with an increased risk for cardiac dysfunction and heart failure itself. Assessment for these alternative etiologies should be part of the evaluation and management of heart failure in adults with CHD.

Table 2
Common heart failure mimics and exacerbating factors among adults with congenital heart disease

Diagnosis or Diagnostic Group	Select Shared Risk Factors, Manifestations, and Associations
Thyroid dysfunction	Trisomy 21, amiodarone, atrial arrhythmia, heart block, and bradycardia
Iron deficiency and anemia	Hypoxemia, anticoagulation, mechanical hemolysis (eg, mechanical valve), blood loss (eg, surgery)
Lung disease	Diaphragm dysfunction, chest wall abnormalities and kyphoscoliosis, airway compression, hyperresponsive airway disease (tetralogy of Fallot with pulmonary atresia)
Chronic kidney disease	Hypoxemia, secondary erythrocytosis, exposure to nephrotoxins, chronic medications, episodic and chronic hypoperfusion
Lymphatic dysfunction	Protein-losing enteropathy, albuminuria, liver disease
Paraganglioma or pheochromocytoma	Hypoxemia, arrhythmias, palpitations, hypertension, anxiety
Obstructive sleep apnea	Trisomy 21, craniofacial malformations
Venous obstruction	Baffle obstruction (Mustard/Senning, Fontan), edema
Liver disease	High-output heart failure, ascites, edema

In addition, CHD is associated with an increased prevalence of psychiatric diagnosis and psychological manifestations. Symptoms may overlap with heart failure, especially fatigue and dyspnea, as well as with arrhythmia or other cardiovascular processes (eg, chest pain). Distinguishing symptoms due to psychological distress can be challenging. However, psychological care is central to CHD care and is crucial to avoid unnecessary and potentially harmful testing and intervention while facilitating appropriate, effective interventions [24] Further, psychiatric and psychological challenges are associated with a markedly increased risk for heart failure and adverse outcomes. One paper found that adults with CHD and a clinical diagnosis of depression had a biomarker phenotype associated with heart failure (higher NT-proBNP and C-reactive peptide) as well as a 3-fold increased risk for mortality.[25]

SUMMARY

With longer survival for those with even the most severe forms of CHD, the consequent aging and increasingly complex CHD population intuitively translates into growing prevalence of heart failure in this population. Defining and managing heart failure in adults with CHD presents challenges due to heterogeneous pathophysiology, atypical manifestations, and commonly coexisting mimics. Care requires a nuanced approach based on individual pathophysiology, appreciating the complexity of hemodynamics status and the centrality of noncardiac contributors, from the lymphatic system to psychosocial factors to the potential for iatrogenic exacerbation of heart failure. Integrating knowledge from pediatric and adult medicine is necessary to deliver optimal care and the best possible outcomes, with an eye toward flexible, experienced clinical judgment rather than dogmatic, algorithmic decision making. As we develop a greater understanding of both CHD and heart failure, our approaches to diagnosis, classification, and management will need to evolve, ensuring that our care is as multifaceted and individual as the patients we serve.

DISCLOSURE

No disclosures related to the topic of this article.

REFERENCES

1. Bozkurt B, Coats AJ, Tsutsui H, et al. Universal Definition and Classification of Heart Failure: A Report of the Heart Failure Society of America, Heart Failure Association of the European Society of Cardiology, Japanese Heart Failure Society and Writing Committee of the Universal Definition of Heart Failure. J Card Fail 2021. :S1071-9164(21)00050-6. doi: 10.1016/j.cardfail.2021.01.022.
2. McLarry J, Broberg C, Opotowsky AR, et al. Defining heart failure in adult congenital heart disease. Prog Pediatr Cardiol 2014;38:3–7.
3. Stout KK, Broberg CS, Book WM, et al. Chronic Heart Failure in Congenital Heart Disease: A Scientific Statement From the American Heart Association. Circulation 2016;133:770–801.
4. Shaddy RE, Boucek MM, Hsu DT, et al. Carvedilol for children and adolescents with heart failure: a randomized controlled trial. JAMA 2007;298:1171–9.
5. Hsu DT, Zak V, Mahony L, et al. Enalapril in infants with single ventricle: results of a multicenter randomized trial. Circulation 2010;122:333–40.
6. Burchill L, Ross HJ, Opotowsky AR. Heart failure in adults with congenital heart disease. In: Jefferies JL, Chang AC, Rossano JW, et al, editors. Heart failure in the child and young adult: from bench to bedside. Academic Press, Elsevier; 2018. p. 331–52.
7. Gallego P, Oliver JM. Medical therapy for heart failure in adult congenital heart disease: does it work? Heart 2020;106:154–62.
8. Norozi K, Wessel A, Alpers V, et al. Incidence and risk distribution of heart failure in adolescents and adults with congenital heart disease after cardiac surgery. Am J Cardiol 2006;97:1238–43.
9. Menachem JN, Opotowsky AR. The art of caring for adults with congenital heart disease in the face of imperfect data. Int J Cardiol 2020;300:141–2.
10. Wessler BS, Kramer DG, Kelly JL, et al. Drug and device effects on peak oxygen consumption, 6-minute walk distance, and natriuretic peptides as predictors of therapeutic effects on mortality in patients with heart failure and reduced ejection fraction. Circ Heart Fail 2011;4:578–88.
11. Cunningham JW, Myhre PL. NT-proBNP Response to Heart Failure Therapies: An Imperfect Surrogate. J Am Coll Cardiol 2021;78:1333–6.
12. Kim SJ, Kwon OD, Han EB, et al. Impact of number of medications and age on adherence to antihypertensive medications: A nationwide population-based study. Medicine 2019;98:e17825.
13. Opotowsky AR. Clinical evaluation and management of pulmonary hypertension in the adult with congenital heart disease. Circulation 2015;131:200–10.
14. Opotowsky AR, Landzberg MJ, Beghetti M. The exceptional and far-flung manifestations of heart failure in Eisenmenger syndrome. Heart Fail Clin 2014;10:91–104.
15. Dimopoulos K, Diller GP, Opotowsky AR, et al. Definition and Management of Segmental Pulmonary Hypertension. J Am Heart Assoc 2018;7.
16. Marcus JT, Gan CT, Zwanenburg JJ, et al. Interventricular mechanical asynchrony in pulmonary arterial

hypertension: left-to-right delay in peak shortening is related to right ventricular overload and left ventricular underfilling. J Am Coll Cardiol 2008;51:750–7.

17. Gelman S. Venous function and central venous pressure: a physiologic story. Anesthesiology 2008;108: 735–48.

18. Veldtman GR, Opotowsky AR, Wittekind SG, et al. Cardiovascular adaptation to the Fontan circulation. Congenit Heart Dis 2017;12:699–710.

19. Bradley EA, Cai A, Cheatham SL, et al. Mustard baffle obstruction and leak - How successful are percutaneous interventions in adults? Prog Pediatr Cardiol 2015;39:157–63.

20. Itkin M, Rockson SG, Burkhoff D. Pathophysiology of the Lymphatic System in Patients With Heart Failure: JACC State-of-the-Art Review. J Am Coll Cardiol 2021;78:278–90.

21. Fudim M, Salah HM, Sathananthan J, et al. Lymphatic Dysregulation in Patients With Heart Failure: JACC Review Topic of the Week. J Am Coll Cardiol 2021;78:66–76.

22. Atton G, Gordon K, Brice G, et al. The lymphatic phenotype in Turner syndrome: an evaluation of nineteen patients and literature review. Eur J Hum Genet 2015;23:1634–9.

23. Mackie AS, Veldtman GR, Thorup L, et al. Plastic Bronchitis and Protein-Losing Enteropathy in the Fontan Patient: Evolving Understanding and Emerging Therapies. Can J Cardiol 2022;38: 988–1001.

24. Kovacs AH, Brouillette J, Ibeziako P, et al. Psychological outcomes and interventions for individuals with congenital heart disease: a scientific statement from the American Heart Association. Circulation: Cardiovascular Quality and Outcomes 2022;15: e000110.

25. Carazo MR, Kolodziej MS, DeWitt ES, et al. Prevalence and Prognostic Association of a Clinical Diagnosis of Depression in Adult Congenital Heart Disease: Results of the Boston Adult Congenital Heart Disease Biobank. J Am Heart Assoc 2020;9: e014820.

Medical Therapy and Monitoring in Adult Congenital Heart Disease Heart Failure

Jeremy Nicolarsen, MD[a,*], James Mudd, MD[b], Andrew Coletti, MD[b]

KEYWORDS

- Adult congenital heart disease • Heart failure • Heart failure therapies • Follow-up • Fontan
- Systemic right ventricle • Eisenmenger syndrome

KEY POINTS

- Heart failure (HF) is a common problem for patients with adult congenital heart disease (ACHD).
- Standard HF therapies have been less well-studied in patients with ACHD with HF, and their use is often driven by small studies and expert opinion.
- Certain groups of patients with ACHD have a higher prevalence of HF—single functional ventricle (Fontan), systemic right ventricle, Eisenmenger syndrome, and severe valvular heart disease.
- Long-term follow-up of ACHD HF requires an understanding of congenital heart defects and their palliative interventions and surgeries, regular surveillance testing, comprehensive team-based care, and clear communication between patients and providers.

BACKGROUND

The prevalence and impact of heart failure (HF) in adults with congenital heart disease (CHD) are increasing every year. At least 20% of hospital admissions of patients with adult congenital heart disease (ACHD) in the United States are for a primary diagnosis of HF.[1] Among the many comorbidities patients with ACHD face, HF impacts their quality and length of life in meaningful ways, and symptoms of HF are often reported as significant detractors of quality of life.[2] In addition, patients with ACHD with HF use health care resources in a much more significant way than their peers without HF,[3–5] and death from HF continues to lead all other causes of mortality in patients with ACHD.[6] Although patients with single functional ventricle physiology, systemic right ventricles (RVs), severe pulmonary arterial

hypertension and Eisenmenger syndrome (ES), and severe valvular heart disease (such as repaired tetralogy of Fallot) continue to experience a greater burden of HF compared with their peers with less severe CHD,[7,8] HF continues to impact all types of patients with ACHD, with many experiencing HF symptoms at some point in their lives.[9]

Most patients with CHD are expected to reach adulthood and are now living longer thanks to innovation in the operative and interventional arenas, improved awareness and organization of care, and an expansion of the use and availability of advanced HF therapies, such as mechanical circulatory support and transplantation. Although ACHD care has significantly improved in these areas over the past several decades, much remains unknown and unvalidated for medical therapy for HF. Medical therapies for left ventricular systolic and/or diastolic dysfunction in patients

[a] Providence Adult and Teen Congenital Heart Program (PATCH), Providence Sacred Heart Medical Center and Children's Hospital, 101 West 8th Avenue, Suite 4300, Spokane, WA 99204, USA; [b] Center for Advanced Heart Disease and Transplantation, Providence Spokane Heart Institute, 62 West 7th Avenue, Suite 232, Spokane, WA 99204, USA
* Corresponding author.
E-mail address: jeremy.nicolarsen@providence.org

Heart Failure Clin 20 (2024) 137–146
https://doi.org/10.1016/j.hfc.2023.12.002
1551-7136/24/© 2023 Elsevier Inc. All rights reserved.

without CHD have greatly expanded in recent years, particularly with the addition of therapies such as angiotensin receptor/neprilysin inhibitors (ARNIs) and sodium glucose cotransport-2 (SGLT2) inhibitors,[10] but the same gains have not been realized for patients with ACHD with HF. Studies on HF therapies in patients with ACHD are small in number and size, with few notable positive results, especially for patients with systemic right ventricular failure or single functional ventricles. Although these new medications have revolutionized HF care for patients with left ventricle (LV) failure, they remain unstudied in patients with ACHD, impacting reimbursement, availability, and usage.

Management of patients with ACHD with HF relies on a variety of approaches, understanding the nuanced types of HF in a heterogeneous population, and willingness to try therapies such as ARNIs and SGLT2 inhibitors in a data-free zone. ACHD and HF cardiologists who manage HF in these patients must do so with flexibility not necessarily seen in other areas of cardiovascular care. There must be an understanding of a wide range of underlying defects and the various palliative surgeries and interventions used to treat CHD, as well as an awareness of the natural history and expected outcomes a patient with ACHD may experience in his/her lifetime. Medical therapy for ACHD HF is only part of the story; managing HF in this patient population also requires a willingness of the ACHD and HF provider to regularly communicate with the patient, a thorough approach to identifying related diseases, such as liver and renal dysfunction, and a team-based approach to care. This comprehensive and longitudinal follow-up is critical to improve outcomes for patients with ACHD with HF.

MEDICAL THERAPY

There are 4 types of patients with ACHD who are most likely to develop HF and have the greatest morbidity and mortality among their peers with CHD: those with single functional ventricle physiology (typically palliated with a series of surgeries ending in a total cavopulmonary anastomosis [Fontan]), systemic RVs (d-Transposition of the great arteries palliated with an atrial switch operation [Mustard or Senning] or congenitally corrected transposition [CC-TGA]), severe pulmonary arterial hypertension and ES, and severe valvular heart disease.

Single Functional Ventricle Physiology

In complex CHD with one dominant systemic ventricle, such as tricuspid atresia or hypoplastic left heart syndrome (HLHS), patients are often, but not universally, palliated with a series of surgeries ending in a total cavopulmonary anastomosis, in which the entirety of the systemic venous return is passively routed to the lungs, and pulmonary venous blood returns to the heart and is distributed to the body by the systemic ventricle. These palliative surgeries have undergone a series of modifications since the results of the original Fontan procedure were first published in 1971,[11] including variations of the atriopulmonary connection and lateral tunnel Fontan. The current era of Fontan palliation involves a superior cavopulmonary anastomosis (bidirectional Glenn anastomosis) connecting the superior vena cava to the cranial side of the right pulmonary artery (RPA) and the use of an extracardiac Gor-Tex conduit connecting the inferior vena cava to the underside (caudal side) of the RPA. Colloquially known as the "Glenn" and "Fontan" stages, these palliative surgeries typically occur at 3 to 6 months of age (Glenn) and 2 to 3 years of age (Fontan), both usually following some neonatal palliative surgery, such as a Norwood surgery for HLHS or an atriopulmonary shunt for cases of right heart hypoplasia with inadequate pulmonary blood flow.

Although there are many variations in these surgeries and their timing, they essentially result in a shared physiology that depends on slightly elevated central venous pressure; low pulmonary artery pressure and pulmonary vascular resistance (PVR); a lack of Fontan, Glenn, or pulmonary artery stenoses; a compliant systemic ventricle with low filling pressures and adequate systemic ventricular function (systolic and diastolic); and minimal valvular heart disease. Derangements in one or several of these areas can accelerate comorbid conditions that often affect adult Fontan patients, such as liver fibrosis and cirrhosis, arrhythmias, kidney disease, protein-losing enteropathy, and plastic bronchitis. Fontan patients may also require arrhythmia ablation, cardiac implantable electric devices, interventional cardiac catheterizations, and even more surgery if valvular heart disease is significant. Without intervention or medical therapy, Fontan patients are expected to face decisions about transplantation (heart or combined organ transplant, often heart-liver) or palliative care, often by the fifth or sixth decade, or earlier if comorbidities exist.[12]

Medical therapy to treat Fontan patients is highly nuanced, and there is a lack of randomized trial data to guide management. Therapies targeted at lowering pulmonary artery pressures, such as phosphodiesterase-5 inhibitors (PDE5i) or endothelin receptor antagonists (ERA),[13–15] and others address afterload reduction and ventricular remodeling, such as beta-blockers, angiotensin-converting enzyme inhibitors (ACEi), angiotensin receptor blockers (ARB), and mineralocorticoid receptor inhibitors (MRA).[16] Finally, there is hope ARNIs and SGLT2 inhibitors may have some benefit in systemic ventricular failure in Fontan patients, but data remain limited.

Pulmonary vasodilator therapy in Fontan patients has been an area of interest for many. The FUEL trial (Fontan Udenafil Exercise Longitudinal), one of the largest phase III clinical trials to date, evaluated the efficacy of PDE5i therapy in adolescent and young adult Fontan patients; treatment with udenafil (87.5 mg twice daily) was not associated with an improvement in oxygen consumption at peak exercise over placebo, the primary outcome of the study.[14] There were improvements, however, in other measures of exercise performance at the anaerobic threshold, and the drug was well tolerated.[14] Another large phase III clinical trial evaluating ERA therapy in Fontan patients, the RUBATO trial, has completed data collection but has yet to publish results. Prepublication data presented at the 2022 European Society of Cardiology Congress suggest macitentan (10 mg once daily) did not meet the RUBATO trial's primary efficacy endpoint of improvement of peak oxygen consumption at 16 weeks compared with placebo.[17]

Because of the lack of data on effective medical therapy in Fontan patients, if HF medications are used at all, they are often not started until there are known physiologic abnormalities, such as elevated pulmonary artery, Fontan, or filling pressures by hemodynamic cardiac catheterization, or progressive symptoms. Further adding to the challenge of treating these patients is their substantial heterogeneity. Even the anatomy of the systemic ventricle seems to be important,[18,19] with systemic LV possibly benefiting more from standard HF therapy.

Systemic Right Ventricle

The RV is the systemic (or subaortic) ventricle in patients with d-Transposition of the great arteries (d-TGA) palliated with the atrial switch surgery (Mustard or Senning) or in CC-TGA (also known as L-TGA with ventricular inversion). In each of these cases, the RV is faced with a lifetime of systemic pressures and different loading conditions than is typical for a subpulmonary RV, thus inciting remodeling (hypertrophy and chamber enlargement) that may eventually become problematic. The health of the systemic RV is highly variable, but most patients with d-TGA treated with atrial switch surgery or CC-TGA will likely face systemic RV failure in their fifth to sixth decade, especially those with concomitant tricuspid valve dysfunction.[20,21]

In d-TGA, the cardiac chambers are positioned normally, but the aorta is rightward and anterior to the pulmonary artery and originates from the RV. Systemic venous blood enters the right atrium (RA) but is then directed out the aorta having not been oxygenated in the lungs; thus, intracardiac mixing at the atrial level through an atrial septal defect (and often, ventricular level through a ventricular septal defect) is necessary for oxygenated pulmonary venous return to the body, but at the cost of cyanosis. The Mustard and Senning surgeries, both first used in the 1960s,[22,23] involve the creation of an intra-atrial baffle (wall) to redirect systemic venous blood from the RA to the subpulmonary LV and pulmonary venous blood from the left atrium (LA) to the systemic RV. Adults repaired with this *atrial* switch can develop stenosis of the systemic and/or pulmonary venous portions of the baffle, atrial arrhythmias such as intra-atrial reentrant tachyarrhythmias or sinus node dysfunction, and systemic RV dysfunction. In most cases, this surgical palliation has been largely abandoned because of this myriad of complications and has been supplanted by the *arterial* switch operation (ASO), a neonatal surgery first described in 1976.[24] ASO involves transection of the aorta and pulmonary artery followed by anastomosis to their appropriate ventricle (aorta to LV and pulmonary artery to RV) and translocation of the coronary arteries to the *neoaorta*, thus creating a physiologically appropriate systemic *LV*. The ASO avoids systemic RV failure and has a lower burden of atrial arrhythmias; however, neoaortic dilatation, ostial coronary compression, supravalvar aorta or pulmonary artery stenosis, and/or branch pulmonary artery stenosis can occur. Still, these complications occur less frequently and are generally less significant than those occurring after the Mustard or Senning surgery.

In CC-TGA (or L-TGA with ventricular inversion), the atrial anatomy is normal, the ventricles are L-looped with the morphologic LV on the right and the morphologic RV on the left, and the aorta is left and anterior (to the pulmonary artery) and originates from a *systemic* RV. Systemic venous blood flow returns to the RA normally and then crosses the mitral valve to enter the subpulmonary LV, followed by the pulmonary arteries. Pulmonary venous blood flow returning to the heart enters the LA, followed by the RV after passing through the tricuspid valve, and is then pumped into the aorta. CC-TGA allows for physiologically appropriate circulation in that systemic venous return is directed to the lungs for oxygenation, and systemic arterial blood flow is therefore adequately oxygenated; however, this comes at the cost of the RV remaining the systemic ventricle. Because the RV is not aptly suited for systemic cardiac output, systemic RV enlargement and dysfunction are common as is systemic tricuspid regurgitation. This inefficient system can lead to significant comorbidities, including HF and complications from low cardiac output.

An important concept in systemic RV failure is the altered morphology and muscle fiber structure of the RV. Unlike the bullet-shaped LV with circumferential and longitudinal muscle fibers that work in concert to maximize contraction, the RV has an altered array of muscle fibers that are not equipped to maintain the same degree of contraction and perform well at systemic pressures.[25] In addition, the abnormal shape of the RV and variable loading conditions (volume, pressure, or both, depending on CHD type) predisposes the RV to early ventricular failure in some cases. For these reasons, it is thought the response of the RV to medical therapy may not be the same as the systemic LV in structurally normal hearts. Although the renin-angiotensin-aldosterone system (RAAS) is likely upregulated in systemic RV failure and using medical therapy to target this system may be helpful, the response of the RV myocardium to standard HF therapy is thought to be less optimal.[26]

Severe Pulmonary Arterial Hypertension and Eisenmenger Syndrome

When left-to-right shunt lesions, such as atrial or ventricular septal defects, patent ductus arteriosus, or partial anomalous pulmonary venous return, go unrepaired, prolonged and excessive pulmonary blood flow can lead to pulmonary vascular changes that increase pulmonary vascular resistance (PVR) to the point of shunt reversal. This transition to right-to-left shunting, or ES,[27] is often associated with cyanosis, clubbing of the digits, iron-deficient erythrocytosis, hemoptysis, thrombosis, and stroke.[28] The pulmonary vasculature smooth muscle is hypertrophied, thereby increasing PVR, which in turn increases RV afterload and can lead to RV chamber enlargement, hypertrophy, and dysfunction progressing to clinical right HF. Patients with ES have diminished exercise tolerance[29] and shortened lifespans and often die from one or several of the complications outlined above.[30]

Medical therapy in ES is limited and primarily targets RV afterload reduction through pulmonary vasodilator therapies. Two ERAs, bosentan and macitentan, have been studied in large clinical trials thus far. The BREATHE-5 trial (Bosentan Randomized Trial of Endothelin Antagonist Therapy-5) showed improved 6-minute walk distance and hemodynamics (by heart catheterization) with bosentan over placebo.[31] However, the MAESTRO trial (Macitentan in Eisenmenger Syndrome to Restore Exercise Capacity) did not show a benefit of macitentan over placebo at improving peak oxygen consumption at 16 weeks.[32] It should be noted that in a hemodynamic substudy of the MAESTRO trial, NT-proBNP and PVR index improved with macitentan.[32]

Outside of pulmonary vasodilators, other therapies for ES are intended to treat the comorbidities that arise with this condition, such as iron supplementation for iron-deficient erythrocytosis, supplemental oxygen for hypoxemia-related symptoms (although supplemental O_2 has no impact on disease progression or mortality), and oral anticoagulation for patients with thrombosis.[33] Elective phlebotomy is no longer indicated in most cases and should only be used for patients with a hematocrit greater than 65 and symptoms of hyperviscosity.[34]

Severe Valvular Heart Disease

Severe valvular heart disease in ACHD is common,[35] especially in older patients with ACHD.[36] In most cases, transcatheter or surgical valve intervention is an option to improve valve hemodynamics and related HF. However, not all patients are candidates for interventional or surgical valve therapy owing to excessive procedural or operative risk, challenges with vascular access, or availability of local or regional expertise. In these cases, and for most patients who would benefit from delayed palliation of valvular heart disease (a young patient with tetralogy of Fallot who will need multiple pulmonary valves in his/her lifetime, for example), medical therapy may be used to try to maintain the health of native or prosthetic valves, although data to support this are lacking.[37]

Intuitively, pulmonary or systemic afterload-reducing medications should help regurgitant valves, but studies have not shown a significant impact in this area.[37] A better focus of medical therapy may be on the ventricular myocardium, particularly in cases of LV enlargement/dysfunction with secondary mitral regurgitation, with medications such as beta-blockers, RAAS inhibitors (ACEi, ARB, MRA, ARNI), and SGLT2 inhibitors, by slowing the ventricular remodeling that occurs in valvular heart disease and maintaining adequate cardiac output, or by decongestive medications like loop diuretics, to improve myocardial size/function or leaflet coaptation.[38] Practically, these medications are used when valvular heart disease has already impacted ventricular systolic or diastolic function and/or has led to symptoms, but there is not yet enough evidence to support the prophylactic use of HF medications in these patients. Often, these medications are added while interventional or surgical therapies are being arranged.

The Future of Heart Failure Medical Therapy for Patients with Adult Congenital Heart Disease

Medical therapy for each of these subtypes of complex CHD varies slightly, and large clinical trials supporting their use are few. Often, the choice of medical therapy for HF in complex CHD relies on small case series, retrospective multicenter reviews, and anecdotal and expert opinion. However, there is increasing interest in the study of HF medications in patients with CHD of all ages and in more meaningful ways. PANORAMA-HF, for example, is the largest prospective study of *pediatric* patients with HF owing to left ventricular systolic dysfunction with biventricular physiology and aims to evaluate the efficacy and safety of sacubitril/valsartan versus enalapril.[39] If clinical research in CHD HF can be organized in such a way as this study and if enrollment can be successful for pediatric patients, the future is bright for understanding HF therapy in ACHD.

FOLLOW-UP AND MONITORING

Regardless of medical, interventional, and surgical therapies, most cases of HF in patients with ACHD involve slow progression to advanced HF requiring mechanical circulatory support, transplant, or palliative care and hospice.[40] There can be many years of stability once HF symptoms begin, and some patients experience periods of improvement with the initiation of medications or interventions, such as valve repair/replacement. However, as with HF in patients without CHD, there are periods of acute worsening requiring hospitalization or adjustment of therapy, along with a gradual decline in functional status and quality of life.[40] These periods of decompensation, or *HF events*, may be triggered by arrhythmia, medicine nonadherence, dietary indiscretion, or exacerbation of other comorbid conditions occurring without warning.

Follow-up and monitoring during this variably long period of gradual HF worsening is important and requires regular surveillance office visits and diagnostic testing, as well as and an awareness of the signs of an impending HF event, such as rapid weight gain, decreased response to diuretic therapy, and/or increased dyspnea or palpitations. Patients and families need to be educated about the signs and symptoms of HF and that

progression of disease is expected. However, successful management of ACHD HF is possible with a close relationship between the patient and the ACHD or HF team, and a commitment by both sides (patient and provider) to communicate effectively to minimize the frequency or impact of HF events.

Diagnostic Testing and Surveillance in Adult Congenital Heart Disease Heart Failure

Surveillance testing in patients with ACHD with HF should be comprehensive and occur on a regular basis (**Fig. 1**). At a minimum, it should include physical examination, electrocardiography to screen for occult arrhythmia, echocardiography to assess cardiac and valve function, and laboratory evaluation to monitor organ function and trend HF biomarkers. Additional testing, such as cardiac MRI, cardiac computed tomography with angiography, and cardiac catheterization, should be used as well, especially when HF worsens, or HF events have no apparent cause. Six-minute walk testing or cardiopulmonary exercise testing will help objectively monitor functional status, evaluate response to therapies or interventions, and guide discussion about prognosis. Finally, in cases in which HF management is challenging and patients struggle to maintain euvolemia, ambulatory pulmonary artery pressure monitoring with implantable hemodynamic monitors, such as the CardioMEMS HF System (Abbott Medical, Atlanta, GA), can alert providers of hemodynamic changes that warrant a therapy change to prevent an HF exacerbation.[41] Regardless of the type of testing used for HF surveillance, the ACHD or HF provider should communicate with the patient that consistent follow-up and testing are critical to identify changes before they result in an HF event or HF worsening and that each of these diagnostic tests plays a different role in comprehensive evaluation monitoring.

As patients with ACHD with HF progressively decline in functional status or develop worsening symptoms or diagnostic testing, the frequency of follow-up should invariably increase. The 2018 American College of Cardiology/American Heart Association ACHD Guidelines outline surveillance testing and frequency by assigning an anatomic complexity and physiologic classification to most patients who will be seen in an ACHD or HF office.[42] These surveillance plans can be used to guide decisions about the frequency of follow-up and timing of diagnostic testing and serve as a useful tool when communicating with patients and insurers about the need for certain testing. Most patients with moderate anatomic complexity

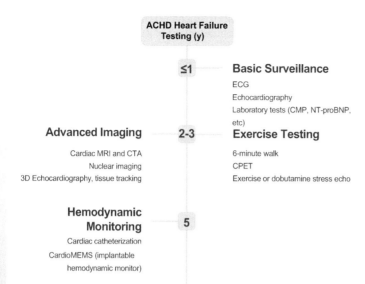

Fig. 1. Surveillance testing should be comprehensive and occur on a regular basis, as suggested here. Deviations from these frequencies are expected, depending on HF severity and disease complexity. The 2018 American College of Cardiology/American Heart Association ACHD Guidelines outline testing intervals for most all CHD types and physiologic complexity, but a general approach like this could be applied to all patients with ACHD with HF. 3D, three dimensional; CMP, comprehensive metabolic panel; CPET, cardiopulmonary exercise testing; CTA, computed tomographic angiography; ECG, electrocardiogram; NT-proBNP, N-terminal b-type natriuretic peptide.

and class C or D physiologic state (the worst 2 physiologic classes) are seen at least once a year, and severely complex patients with advanced disease, class IIID, should visit their ACHD or HF provider every 3 to 6 months. Of course, deviation from these guideline recommendations is expected, especially for patients with rapidly progressive HF, but the surveillance plans outlined have significantly improved the organization of HF care for the patient with ACHD.

Communication Between Patient with Adult Congenital Heart Disease and Provider

Patients with ACHD with HF often differ in their experiences and interactions with cardiac care from those who develop HF later in life (acquired heart disease). Except for late diagnoses of CHD in adulthood, most adult patients with CHD were once *children* with heart disease and have been visiting cardiology offices and undergoing cardiac testing for years before their development of HF. Most patients with CHD (and their parents or caretakers) have experienced sudden changes in health and unexpected hospitalizations or interventions that come with this complex and nuanced form of heart disease. Their understanding of and relationship with heart disease likely have impacted their assessment of the severity of their condition, and patients with ACHD who develop HF may have widely different views on the impact of HF on their lives.

Many patients with ACHD have never known "normal" and may not recognize gradual progression of heart disease,[43] instead thinking that worsening dyspnea might be expected, secondary to weight gain or deconditioning, or simply because of "getting older." In addition, patients with ACHD typically have lower exercise capacity than their peers[44–46] and may be more sedentary and may not notice a gradual decline in exercise tolerance. Whether their assessment of their health status is appropriate or not, patients with ACHD may not proactively communicate with their ACHD or HF provider about subtle changes in symptoms. Some may be stoic and tolerate significant symptoms and fail to recognize these changes for what they may be, such as an impending HF event that might be preventable with a change in therapy. Conversely, some patients with ACHD have experienced cardiac decompensation in their past or may be less informed about what HF symptoms really look like, and they may live with heightened fear or awareness of slight changes in how they feel and therefore contact their ACHD or HF team frequently. This can create caregiver burden and underappreciation of symptom reports when there truly is a change in clinical status. The key for either of these types of patients with ACHD, the nonreporter or the overreporter, is that ACHD and HF providers and teams communicate clearly about the expectations of what to expect from HF and remain available and responsive to calls and messages from patients, using these touch points as opportunities for education and trust/rapport development.

Early Referral for Transplant Evaluation or Palliative Care

There comes a point where the frequency or duration of HF events or hospitalizations increases, comorbid conditions such as renal failure complicate management, or symptoms worsen to a point that significantly impacts quality of life and a clear trajectory of increased morbidity and mortality is evident. That is when patients with HF with ACHD and their providers need to decide whether to move forward with evaluation for heart (or combined organ) transplantation or transition to less aggressive care and focus on palliation. Except for a terminal hospitalization, this moment is not usually defined by a specific event, but rather a series of setbacks from which emergence to a prior physiologic and clinical state appears unachievable. Although some argue this is the time for referral to an advanced disease and heart transplant (AHDT) program, the case should be made to begin conversations about goals of care and transplantation much earlier in an ACHD patient's HF course. Although not all patients with ACHD will experience HF in their lifetime and mortality occurs for a variety of reasons, there should be an expanding role and earlier involvement of AHDT and palliative care teams in the care of these patients (**Fig. 2**).

For some conditions, such as the four described above, discussions about transplantation and palliative care should consistently occur between patients and ACHD providers, and they should start years before referral. Many times, the patient with ACHD will appreciate a forewarning of what is to come, and clear communication on this topic will aid in financial and estate planning, encourage discussions among families about advanced directives, and help patients and their families prioritize life activities. Conversations about prognosis, setting expectations around transplant evaluation and timing, and honest discussions about the current and future impact of HF on one's life are critical. Finally, although early referral to AHDT or palliative care teams is important, this should be done sensitively, as it can elicit a change in an ACHD patient's perception of their own health; patients should be informed and not disabled by communication about prognosis.

THE IMPORTANCE OF COLLABORATIVE CARE

Management of the patient with ACHD with HF is a team sport. Although the ACHD provider and support group (nurse coordinator, social worker, and so forth) are often on the frontlines guiding care, there is a point when an AHDT team needs to be involved, if only to confirm that current

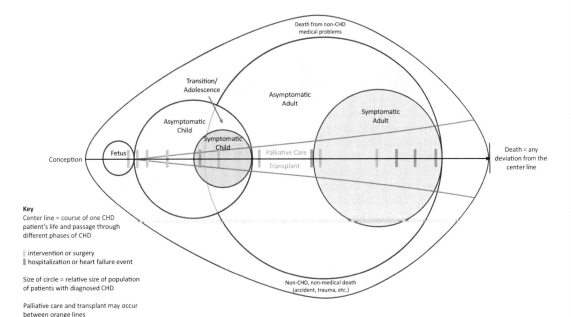

Fig. 2. The course of a patient's life with CHD (*center line*) through the potential stages of CHD (*circles*). Not every stage will be entered with death (migration away from the *center line*) occurring at any stage or unrelated to CHD. Patients enter and leave stages in different ways—some with a fetus diagnosis of CHD; others diagnosed as children or adults. The size of the CHD stage reflects the relative size of the population in that stage. Events along one's life may include interventions or surgeries (*blue lines*) or hospitalizations or HF events (*orange lines*). Some patients may experience no events, while others may experience many events (as shown). Palliative care and transplant (heart or combined organ) may occur at any stage but increase with age and symptoms. In coming years, with the exception of pediatric circles, the size of fetus and adult circles, distance between orange palliative care and transplant lines, and length of the center line should all increase and, possibly, there will be less blue and orange events with improvements in technology and health care.

management strategies are appropriate. This not only helps the ACHD provider ensure his or her therapeutic plans are sound but also enhances the message to the patient that comprehensive, team-based care is being provided by various providers with different expertise. Although the AHDT provider is often the most knowledgeable about the many and varied HF medical therapies available to date and involving him/her early in ACHD HF care is important, the ACHD provider may have a better understanding of the nuanced care necessary for each CHD and have some insight into an individual patient's goals and wishes because of the length of their relationship before HF. Therefore, ACHD and AHDT providers should complement each other, learn from one another, and together improve the care of the patient with ACHD with HF.

The relationship between the ACHD and AHDT teams and their providers and staff should be cultivated, and opportunities should be created for the 2 teams to *share* the care of patients with HF with ACHD, especially as this patient population grows. This can come in the form of multidisciplinary patient review conferences, as is done by each team for their own patients, or in regularly scheduled didactic meetings. In addition, there may be opportunities for joint rounding on inpatients or collaborative clinics for stable outpatients with ACHD with HF. The authors of this paper have created a regular multidisciplinary clinic for HF patients with HF with ACHD that is attended by ACHD and AHDT teams, as well as palliative care providers and the ACHD social worker. Patients and their families periodically attend this afternoon-long clinic and meet with each of the groups in turn and in the same physical space, thus allowing for the creation of a comprehensive and updated plan agreed to by all parties. An ACHD-HF multidisciplinary clinic begins with a "prebrief" on each patient and opportunity for education, followed by a "debrief" at the end of the afternoon, and plans are organized for rapid implementation.

Regardless of the mechanism for ACHD and AHDT teams to collaborate in the care of patients with HF with ACHD, this advanced degree of care for the sickest of patients relies heavily on effective communication (patient to provider and provider to provider), mutual respect among all parties, a willingness to educate and improve each other's care, and an organizational structure that keeps the patient central and which optimizes the care he or she receives. Patients with CHD are cared for throughout their lives in this expansive way and by multiple providers (cardiologists of all types, CHD surgeons, inpatient and outpatient nurses, consulting subspecialists, and so forth), so why should it be any different for a patient with ACHD with HF? Arguably, care at this stage in an ACHD patient's life should be the most organized and collaborative yet.

SUMMARY

Patients with CHD are not just surviving to adulthood at increasing rates, they are living longer and undergoing palliative medical, interventional, and surgical therapies that will carry them into increasingly older ages. HF in the patient with ACHD is no longer an occasional challenge for the ACHD provider, but a common occurrence. Similarly, the AHDT provider may be noticing an increasing number of patients with ACHD referred for HF management and/or formal transplant evaluation.

The use of medical therapies for ACHD HF remains a data-free, or *data-light*, zone, especially for patients with severely complex disease, such as single functional ventricle, systemic RV, ES, or severe valvular heart disease. However, understanding of the pathophysiology and therapeutic aspects of ACHD HF must continue to be expanded, diagnostic testing and surveillance must be standardized, and the infrastructure to support collaborative care among all providers caring for this growing and challenging group of patients must evolve.

CLINICS CARE POINTS

- As survival for patients with adult congenital heart disease improves, so too will the prevalence of heart failure.

- Well-studied and highly tailored medical therapies do not exist for patients with heart failure with adult congenital heart disease.

- Heart failure is more common in certain types of patients with adult congenital heart disease, particularly those with functional single ventricles, systemic right ventricles, Eisenmenger syndrome, and severe valvular heart disease.

- Heart failure management for the patient with adult congenital heart disease requires regular comprehensive cardiac testing, team-based collaborative care between adult congenital heart disease, heart failure, and palliative care providers, and frequent communication with patients and their families.

DISCLOSURE

The authors have a consulting agreement with Medtronic.

REFERENCES

1. Rodriguez FH, Moodie DS, Parekh DR, et al. Adult congenital heart disease heart failure. Congenit Hear Dis 2013;8(6):513–9.

2. Ly R, Karsenty C, Amedro P, et al. Health-related quality of life and its association with outcomes in adults with congenital heart disease and heart failure: insight from FRESH-ACHD registry. J Am Hear Assoc: Cardiovasc Cerebrovasc Dis 2023;12(8):e027819.

3. Burchill LJ, Gao L, Kovacs AH, et al. Hospitalization trends and health resource use for adult congenital heart disease–related heart failure. J Am Hear Assoc 2018;7(15):e008775.

4. Agarwal S, Sud K, Menon V. Nationwide hospitalization trends in adult congenital heart disease across 2003–2012. J Am Hear Assoc 2016;5(1):e002330.

5. Burstein DS, Rossano JW, Griffis H, et al. Greater admissions, mortality and cost of heart failure in adults with congenital heart disease. Heart 2021; 107(10):807–13.

6. Verheugt CL, Uiterwaal CSPM, van der Velde ET, et al. Mortality in adult congenital heart disease. Eur Hear J 2010;31(10):1220–9.

7. Norozi K, Wessel A, Alpers V, et al. Incidence and risk distribution of heart failure in adolescents and adults with congenital heart disease after cardiac surgery. Am J Cardiol 2006;97(8):1238–43.

8. Guccione P, Iorio FS, Rebonato M, et al. Profiles of heart failure in adolescents and young adults with congenital heart disease. Prog Pediatr Cardiol 2018;51:37–45.

9. Leusveld EM, Kauling RM, Geenen LW, et al. Heart failure in congenital heart disease: management options and clinical challenges. Expert Rev Cardiovasc Ther 2020;18(8):503–16.

10. Tsutsui H. Recent advances in the pharmacological therapy of chronic heart failure: evidence and guidelines. Pharmacol Ther 2022;238(Eur J Heart Fail 23 2021):108185.

11. Fontan F, Baudet E. Surgical repair of tricuspid atresia. Thorax 1971;26(3):240.

12. d'Udekem Y, Iyengar AJ, Cochrane AD, et al. The Fontan procedure. Circulation 2007;116(11_suppl): I-157–64.

13. Constantine A, Dimopoulos K, Jenkins P, et al. Use of pulmonary arterial hypertension therapies in patients with a Fontan circulation: current practice across the United Kingdom. J Am Hear Assoc 2022;11(1):e023035.

14. Goldberg DJ, Zak V, Goldstein BH, et al. Results of the Fontan udenafil exercise longitudinal (FUEL) trial. Circulation 2019;141(8):641–51.

15. Oldenburger NJ, Mank A, Etnel J, et al. Drug therapy in the prevention of failure of the Fontan circulation: a systematic review. Cardiol Young 2016;26(5): 842–50.

16. Wilson TG, Iyengar AJ, Winlaw DS, et al. Use of ACE inhibitors in Fontan: rational or irrational? Int J Cardiol 2016;210:95–9.

17. ESC 365 - The efficacy and safety of macitentan in Fontan-palliated patients: results of the 52-week randomised, placebo-controlled RUBATO trial. Available at: https://esc365.escardio.org/presentation/253540?query=RUBATO%202022. Accessed November 12, 2023.

18. Thornton SW, Meza JM, Prabhu NK, et al. Impact of ventricular dominance on long-term Fontan outcomes: a 25-year single-institution study. Ann Thorac Surg 2022. https://doi.org/10.1016/j.athoracsur.2022.11.039.

19. Ponzoni M, Azzolina D, Vedovelli L, et al. Ventricular morphology of single-ventricle hearts has a significant impact on outcomes after Fontan palliation: a meta-analysis. Eur J Cardio Thorac Surg 2022; 62(6). https://doi.org/10.1093/ejcts/ezac535.

20. Broberg CS, Dissel A van, Minnier J, et al. Long-term outcomes after atrial switch operation for transposition of the great arteries. J Am Coll Cardiol 2022; 80(10):951–63.

21. Egbe AC, Miranda WR, Jain CC, et al. Prognostic implications of progressive systemic ventricular dysfunction in congenitally corrected transposition of great arteries. JACC (J Am Coll Cardiol): Cardiovasc Imaging 2022;15(4):566–74.

22. MUSTARD WT. Successful two-stage correction of transposition of the great vessels. Surgery 1964; 55:469–72.

23. SENNING A. Surgical correction of transposition of the great vessels. Surgery 1959;45(6):966–80.

24. Jatene AD, Fontes VF, Paulista PP, et al. Anatomic correction of transposition of the great vessels. J Thorac Cardiovasc Surg 1976;72(3):364–70.

25. Campanale CM, Scherrer B, Afacan O, et al. Myofiber organization in the failing systemic right ventricle. J Cardiovasc Magn Reson 2020;22(1):49.

26. Lluri G, Aboulhosn J. The systemic right ventricle in adult congenital heart disease: why is it still such a challenge and is there any hope on the horizon? Curr Opin Cardiol 2021;37(1):123–9.

27. Wood P. The Eisenmenger syndrome or pulmonary hypertension week reversed central shunt. Am J Cardiol 1972;30(2):172–4.

28. Chaix M-A, Gatzoulis MA, Diller G-P, et al. Eisenmenger syndrome: a multisystem disorder—do not destabilize the balanced but fragile physiology. Can J Cardiol 2019;35(12):1664–74.

29. Müller J, Hess J, Hager A. Exercise performance and quality of life is more impaired in Eisenmenger syndrome than in complex cyanotic congenital heart

disease with pulmonary stenosis. Int J Cardiol 2009; 150(2):177–81.

30. Hjortshøj CMS, Kempny A, Jensen AS, et al. Past and current cause-specific mortality in Eisenmenger syndrome. Eur Hear J 2017;38(26):2060–7.

31. Galie N, Beghetti M, Gatzoulis MA, et al. Bosentan therapy in patients with Eisenmenger syndrome. Circulation 2006;114(1):48–54.

32. Gatzoulis MA, Landzberg M, Beghetti M, et al. Evaluation of macitentan in patients with Eisenmenger syndrome. Circulation 2018;139(1):51–63.

33. Arvanitaki A, Gatzoulis MA, Opotowsky AR, et al. Eisenmenger syndrome JACC state-of-the-art review. J Am Coll Cardiol 2022;79(12):1183–98.

34. Ammash N, Warnes CA. Cerebrovascular events in adult patients with cyanotic congenital heart disease. J Am Coll Cardiol 1996;28(3):768–72.

35. Graziani F, Iannaccone G, Meucci MC, et al. Impact of severe valvular heart disease in adult congenital heart disease patients. Front Cardiovasc Med 2022;9:983308.

36. Afilalo J, Therrien J, Pilote L, et al. Geriatric congenital heart disease burden of disease and predictors of mortality. J Am Coll Cardiol 2011;58(14):1509–15.

37. Gill H, Chehab O, Allen C, et al. The advantages, pitfalls and limitations of guideline-directed medical therapy in patients with valvular heart disease. Eur J Hear Fail 2021;23(8):1325–33.

38. Nasser R, Assche LV, Vorlat A, et al. Evolution of functional mitral regurgitation and prognosis in medically managed heart failure patients with reduced ejection fraction. JACC (J Am Coll Cardiol): Hear Fail 2017;5(9):652–9.

39. Shaddy R, Burch M, Kantor PF, et al. Baseline characteristics of pediatric patients with heart failure due to systemic left ventricular systolic dysfunction in the PANORAMA-HF trial. Circ: Hear Fail 2023;16(3): e009816.

40. Crossland DS, Bruaene AVD, Silversides CK, et al. Heart failure in adult congenital heart disease: from advanced therapies to end-of-life care. Can J Cardiol 2019;35(12):1723–39.

41. Salavitabar A, Bradley EA, Chisolm JL, et al. Implantable pulmonary artery pressure monitoring device in patients with palliated congenital heart disease: technical considerations and procedural outcomes. Catheter Cardiovasc Interv 2020;95(2): 270–9.

42. Stout KK, Daniels CJ, Aboulhosn JA, et al. 2018 AHA/ACC guideline for the management of adults with congenital heart disease a report of the American College of Cardiology/American Heart Association task force on clinical practice guidelines. J Am Coll Cardiol 2019;73(12):e81–192.

43. Menachem JN, Schlendorf KH, Mazurek JA, et al. Advanced heart failure in adults with congenital heart disease. JACC (J Am Coll Cardiol): Hear Fail 2020;8(2):87–99.

44. Kempny A, Dimopoulos K, Uebing A, et al. Reference values for exercise limitations among adults with congenital heart disease. Relation to activities of daily life—single centre experience and review of published data. Eur Hear J 2012;33(11):1386–96.

45. Dimopoulos K, Diller G-P, Piepoli MF, et al. Exercise intolerance in adults with congenital heart disease. Cardiol Clin 2006;24(4):641–60.

46. Diller G-P, Dimopoulos K, Okonko D, et al. Exercise intolerance in adult congenital heart disease. Circulation 2005;112(6):828–35.

Heart Failure Staging and Indications for Advanced Therapies in Adults with Congenital Heart Disease

Alexander C. Egbe, MD, MPH, MS[a],*, Heidi M. Connolly, MD[b]

KEYWORDS

- Heart failure, • Medical therapy, • Congenital heart disease, • Mortality

KEY POINTS

- Heart failure (HF) is the leading cause of death common in adults with congenital heart disease (CHD).
- Guideline-directed medical therapy for HF is effective in most CHD presents with HF.
- Early recognition of signs of advanced HF and referral for advanced therapies for HF offer the best survival.

INTRODUCTION

Congenital heart disease (CHD) is present in 1% of all live births.[1,2] Although the birth incidence of CHD has not changed over time, there has been a significant improvement in the medical and surgical management resulting in an increased long-term survival of patients with CHD.[1–8] As a result, more than 90% of babies born with CHD in the current era survive to adulthood.[9,10] However, survival of adults with CHD is still significantly less than that of the general population.[5,6,11,12] The median life expectancy of adults with CHD is around 60 years, and heart failure (HF) accounts for more than 60% of deaths in this population.[5,6,11–14] The current review will describe the clinical features of advanced HF, provide an overview of the current therapies for advanced HF, and outline the indications for advanced therapies in adults with CHD presenting with advanced HF.

HEART FAILURE STAGING SCHEME

HF is defined as the inability of the heart to generate adequate cardiac output to meet metabolic demands at normal filling pressures.[15,16]

The American College of Cardiology/American Heart Association (ACC/AHA) guidelines for the management of HF define 4 stages of HF depending on the presence of cardiac remodeling, symptoms, and response to therapy.[17] Stage A HF denotes patients at risk for developing HF but these patients currently do not have cardiac remodeling or HF symptoms. Stage B HF (Pre-HF) denotes patients with cardiac remodeling but without current or earlier history of HF symptoms. Cardiac remodeling is defined as any of the following: structural heart disease, elevated filling pressures, or elevated cardiac biomarkers of myocardial stretch or injury. Stage C HF (symptomatic HF) denotes patients with cardiac remodeling, and current or earlier history of HF symptoms. Stage D HF (advanced HF) denotes patients with marked symptoms of HF requiring recurrent hospitalization despite attempts to optimize guideline-directed medical therapy (GDMT).[18] Based on this HF classification scheme, there is a unidirectional progression of HF from stage A to D (**Fig. 1**).[17,18] The terms "stage D HF" and "advanced HF" describe the same disease phenotype and will be used interchangeably throughout this article.

a Department of Cardiovascular Medicine, Mayo Clinic and Foundation, 200 First Street Southwest, Rochester, MN 55905, USA; b Department of Cardiovascular Medicine, Mayo Clinic, Rochester, MN 55905, USA
* Corresponding author.
E-mail address: egbe.alexander@mayo.edu

Heart Failure Clin 20 (2024) 147–154
https://doi.org/10.1016/j.hfc.2023.12.006
1551-7136/24/© 2024 Elsevier Inc. All rights reserved.

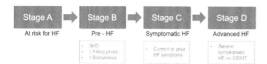

Fig. 1. Flowchart showing the unidirectional progression from stage A to stage D HF. GDMT, guideline-directed medical therapy; HF, heart failure.

CONGENITAL HEART DISEASE STAGING SCHEME

CHD comprise of different structural heart lesions with different anatomic and physiologic characteristics. The native anatomy, type of surgical or transcatheter repair, and current physiology influence the clinical presentation and long-term outcome of the patients.[11,12,19–35] To account for these anatomic and physiologic differences, the

ACC/AHA guidelines for the management of adults with CHD proposed the Anatomic-Physiological (AP) classification scheme.[36] In this classification scheme, the patients are classified into 3 anatomic groups based on the severity of the native lesion (simple CHD, moderately complex CHD, and complex CHD).[36] The physiologic component of the AP classification scheme comprises of 4 disease stages based on symptoms, functional status, aerobic capacity, and end-organ function (**Fig. 2**).[36] In contrast to the HF staging scheme that has unidirectional disease progression (stages A→D), the CHD AP classification scheme allows for a multidirectional disease progression reflecting the natural history of disease or response to therapy (**Fig. 3**). To avoid confusion with the HF classification scheme, we will refer to this classification scheme as CHD AP classification throughout the article.

ACC/AHA Congenital Heart Disease Physiologic Stages

Stage A
NYHA FC I symptoms
No hemodynamic or anatomic sequelae
No arrhythmias
Normal exercise capacity
Normal renal/hepatic/pulmonary function

Stage B
NYHA FC II symptoms
Mild hemodynamic sequelae (mild aortic enlargement, mild ventricular enlargement, mild ventricular dysfunction)
Mild valvular disease
Trivial or small shunt (not hemodynamically significant)
Arrhythmia not requiring treatment
Abnormal objective cardiac limitation to exercise

Stage C
NYHA FC III symptoms
Significant (moderate or greater) valvular disease; moderate or greater ventricular dysfunction (systemic, pulmonic, or both)
Moderate aortic enlargement
Venous or arterial stenosis
Mild or moderate hypoxemia/cyanosis
Hemodynamically significant shunt
Arrhythmias controlled with treatment
Pulmonary hypertension (less than severe)
End-organ dysfunction responsive to therapy[1]

Stage D
NYHA FC IV symptoms
Severe aortic enlargement
Arrhythmias refractory to treatment
Severe hypoxemia (almost always associated with cyanosis)
Severe pulmonary hypertension
Eisenmenger syndrome
Refractory end-organ dysfunction

Fig. 2. Diagnostic criteria for Congenital Heart Disease Physiologic Stages. ACC/AHA, American College of Cardiology/American Heart Association; NYHA, New York heart Association; FC, functional class.

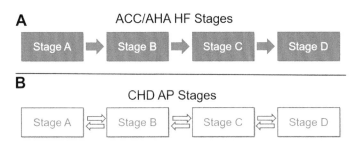

A　　ACC/AHA HF Stages

Stage A ➡ Stage B ➡ Stage C ➡ Stage D

B

CHD AP Stages

Stage A ⇄ Stage B ⇄ Stage C ⇄ Stage D

Fig. 3. Flowchart showing unidirectional disease progression in the ACC/AHA HF staging scheme (A), and multidirectional disease progression in the CHD AP staging scheme (B). ACC/AHA, American College of Cardiology/American Heart Association; AP, anatomic-physiologic; CHD, congenital heart disease.

This multidirectional disease progression is illustrated in a retrospective cohort study of 4588 adults with CHD that had clinical assessment at the time of the first visit to the adult CHD clinic (baseline assessment), and another assessment 3 years later (follow-up assessment).[11] Of the 4588 patients, 3347 (73%) were clinically stable (remained at same CHD AP stage at baseline and follow-up), 855 (19%) had clinical deterioration (advanced to a worse CHD AP stage at follow-up), whereas 386 (8%) had clinical improvement (moved to a lower CHD AP stage at follow-up).[11] Both the CHD AP stage at baseline and temporal change in CHD AP stage during follow-up were associated with all-cause mortality. Using CHD AP stage A as the reference group, the CHD AP stage C and stage D were associated with 19% and 35% increase in the risk of mortality, respectively (**Fig. 4**).[11] Similarly, clinical deterioration was associated with more than 2-fold increase in the risk of mortality, whereas clinical improvement was associated with a 9% reduction in the risk of mortality (see **Fig. 4**).[11]

HEART FAILURE IN CONGENITAL HEART DISEASE: PATHOPHYSIOLOGY AND DISEASE PROGRESSION

Patients with CHD have structural heart disease, and hence by default, they already have stage B HF even in the absence of symptoms. Patients may progress to stage C or D HF over time depending on the underlying disease substrates

(residual or recurrent structural or electrophysiologic lesions), therapeutic interventions (medical, transcatheter, or surgical), and response to therapy.[11,12,37,38] The natural history of HF in CHD is delineated in a retrospective cohort study of 5309 adults with CHD, who received care at the Mayo Clinic Adult Congenital Heart Disease program.[37] At the time of baseline assessment, all patients were in stage B/C HF. However, 432 (8%) patients developed stage D HF during a median follow-up of 4.9 (1.1–7.3) years. The 10-year cumulative incidence of stage D HF was 11% (95% confidence interval [CI] 8–14), corresponding to 1.1% per year.[37] The rate of progression from stage B/C HF to stage D HF varied based on the severity and type of CHD lesion (**Fig. 5**).[37]

OUTCOMES OF STAGE D HEART FAILURE

Studies conducted in patients with HF from acquired heart disease suggest that the onset of stage D HF represents a watershed event in the disease natural history, marked by an exponential increase in the risk of mortality.[18,39] Dunlay and colleagues observed a median survival of 12 months, and a 49% mortality at 1 year after diagnosis of stage D HF in patients with acquired heart disease.[39] Similar dismal outcomes were observed in adults with CHD presenting with stage D HF.[37] Of 432 adults with CHD and stage D HF, 344 (80%) died during a median follow-up of 27 (16–41) months, yielding a mortality rate of 38% per year. Stage D HF was associated with a 6-

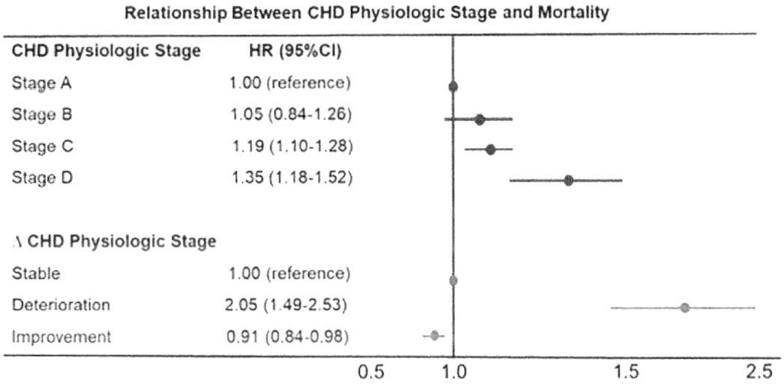

Relationship Between CHD Physiologic Stage and Mortality

CHD Physiologic Stage	HR (95%CI)
Stage A	1.00 (reference)
Stage B	1.05 (0.84-1.26)
Stage C	1.19 (1.10-1.28)
Stage D	1.35 (1.18-1.52)
\ CHD Physiologic Stage	
Stable	1.00 (reference)
Deterioration	2.05 (1.49-2.53)
Improvement	0.91 (0.84-0.98)

0.5　1.0　1.5　2.5

Fig. 4. Forest plot showing the relationship between CHD AP physiologic state and all-cause mortality based on multivariable Cox regression analysis. AP, anatomic-physiologic; CHD, congenital heart disease; CI, confidence interval; HF, heart failure; HR, hazard ratio.

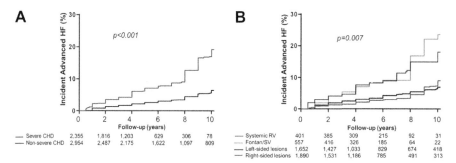

Fig. 5. (*A*) Kaplan–Meier curves comparing cumulative incidence of stage D HF based on CHD severity (*A*) and based on CHD subgroups (*B*). CHD, congenital heart disease; HF, heart failure; RV, right ventricle; SV, single ventricle.

fold increase in the risk of mortality as compared with Stage B/C HF, after adjusting for between-group differences in clinical characteristics (**Fig. 6**).[37] Furthermore, imaging surveillance for recurrent left ventricle (LV) systolic dysfunction should be based on multiple imaging indices including speckle tracking imaging. In a recent study of 193 adults with CHD that underwent serial echocardiograms, the authors showed that LV global longitudinal strain can identify patients at risk for decline in LV ejection fraction and adverse outcomes during follow-up. The study also showed that the patients with absolute LV global longitudinal strain greater than 18% had lower risk of cardiovascular events and decline in LV ejection fraction during follow-up (**Fig. 7**).[33]

MANAGEMENT OF STAGE D HEART FAILURE IN CONGENITAL HEART DISEASE
Overview

Stage D (advanced) HF is characterized by severe HF symptoms that interfere with daily life, and it is often characterized by recurrent hospitalizations despite attempts to optimize GDMT.[17,18] The central goal of HF management is to prevent or delay the onset of stage D HF. However, once a patient develops stage D HF, the risk of mortality

increases exponentially, and the treatment options are limited to advanced therapies for HF.[37] These advanced therapies include intravenous iono-tropic support, mechanical circulatory support, or heart transplantation, and would be addressed in details elsewhere in this review.[17,18]

INDICATIONS FOR ADVANCED THERAPIES FOR HEART FAILURE

Early recognition of the indications for advanced therapies for HF is critical because of the rapid clinical deterioration typically observed at this stage of the disease process. The failure to recognize these indications may delay referral for advanced therapies for HF, which would in turn reduce the odds of survival.

1. Onset of stage D HF.

Stage D HF (advanced HF) is characterized by marked symptoms of HF despite attempts to optimize GDMT. Among adults with CHD, Stage D HF was associated with a 6-fold increase in the risk of mortality as compared with Stage B/C HF, after adjusting for between-group differences in clinical characteristics (see **Fig. 6**). Additionally, clinical deterioration, which is defined as progression to a worse stage of HF, should also prompt a referral for advanced therapies for HF.

2. Recurrent HF hospitalization

Recurrent HF hospitalization, which is defined as more than 1 HF hospitalization within 12 months, is associated with an increased risk of mortality in adults with CHD.[34,35,40] As a result, such patients should be referred for advanced therapies for HF, in order to reduce the risk of mortality observed in such patients.

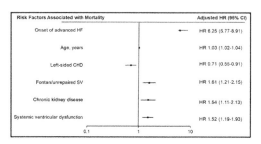

Fig. 6. Forest plot showing the relationship between stage D HF and all-cause mortality based on multivariable Cox regression analysis. CHD, congenital heart disease; CI, confidence interval; HF, heart failure; HR, hazard ratio; SV, single ventricle.

3. Severe biventricular systolic dysfunction

Although CHD diagnosis is typically categorized as predominantly right-sided versus left-sided

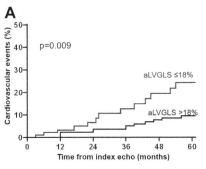 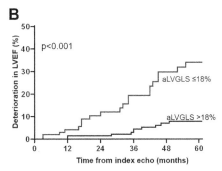

Fig. 7. (A) Kaplan–Meier curves comparing cumulative incidence of cardiovascular events (A), and cumulative incidence of deterioration in aLVEF (B) between patients with aLVGLS greater than 18% versus 18% or greater. LVEF, left ventricular ejection fraction; aLVGLS, absolute left ventricular global longitudinal strain.

lesions, some patients may present with biventricular involvement, and this is a marker of advanced disease.[23,33,41–45] Patients with underlying right-sided lesions (such as tetralogy of Fallot or Ebstein anomaly) presenting with concomitant LV systolic dysfunction, or patients with underlying left-sided lesions (such as coarctation of aorta) presenting with concomitant right ventricular systolic dysfunction have an increased risk of mortality within 5 years.[23,33,41–45] Although there are no standard GDMT for HF for patients with CHD, clinical outcomes studies have demonstrated improved survival using standard GDMT among adults with CHD.[23,33,46] The initial step should, therefore, be to optimize GDMT for HF and then to consider early referral for advanced HF therapy for patients that fail to demonstrate clinical improvement within 6 months of optimal medical therapy.

4. Inoperable valvular heart disease

Surgical and transcatheter therapies remain the first-line treatment of valvular heart disease in patients with CHD.[36,47] However, the presence of concomitant stage D HF, severe left or right ventricular systolic dysfunction, or end-organ dysfunction such as hepatorenal dysfunction are associated with a high risk of early and late mortality following surgical or transcatheter valvular interventions.[37] Patients with valvular heart disease, in the context of these high-risk features, should be referred for advanced therapies for HF, rather than conventional surgical or transcatheter intervention.

5. Severe aerobic or functional impairment

Patients with CHD with New York heart Association class IV symptoms or predicted peak oxygen consumption less than 50% are at risk for cardiovascular and all-cause mortality.[11,48] As a result, patients presenting with these features, in spite of optimal medical therapy, should be referred for advanced therapies for HF.

6. Severe rhythm abnormalities refractory to medical therapy

Patients with CHD are at risk for atrial and ventricular arrhythmias, which in turn, increase the risk for HF, thromboembolic complications, and sudden cardiac death.[42,49,50] The initial therapies for rhythm abnormalities include the use of antiarrhythmic drugs, catheter ablation, and cardiac implantable electronic devices.[42,49,50] However, patients with refractory rhythm abnormalities, in spite of these therapies, should be considered for advance therapies for HF.

7. End-organ dysfunction

End-organ dysfunction such as hepatorenal dysfunction is present in up to 28% of adults with CHD, and this is assisted with all-cause mortality.[51–53] Hepatorenal dysfunction typically does not occur in isolation, and hence, it would not be an absolute indication for advanced therapies for HF.[51–54] However, the presence of hepatorenal dysfunction in the context of stage C HF, should prompt referral for advanced therapies for HF especially if end-organ function does not improve with GDMT for HF.[11,37] Hepatorenal dysfunction typically improves after heart transplant, thereby avoiding the need for multiorgan transplant.[55]

Furthermore, chronic liver disease is common in patients with Fontan palliation, and it is associated with clinical outcomes.[53,56–59] The presence of chronic liver disease such as liver cirrhosis is not an indication for advanced therapies for HF but it is a marker of advanced disease because of the risk of acute liver failure or hepatocellular carcinoma.[60] Hence, Fontan patients with chronic liver disease should be monitored closely and referred for combined heart–liver transplant once these complications occur.[61] Other end-organ dysfunctions that are unique to the Fontan physiology include protein-losing enteropathy and plastic bronchitis.[62,63] There are no standardized therapies for these complications, and hence heart transplant should be considered.

Palliative Care

Unfortunately, not all patients with CHD with stage D HF will be suitable candidates for advanced therapies for HF such as heart transplantation or mechanical circulatory support because of prohibitive factors, such as anatomic complexity, which in turn limits technical feasibility of the procedure, limited donor availability, and severe functional impairment, which reduces the odds of surviving the procedure. As a result, some patients will require palliative care. In the Mayo Clinic cohort, 72 (43%) of the 167 patients with CHD with stage D HF referred for heart transplant evaluation received palliative care because they were not deemed suitable candidates for advanced therapies for HF.[37] This is also consistent with data from other centers suggesting lower probability of receiving an organ transplant in patients with CHD as compared with non-CHD patients.[64] Considering the harsh realities of outcomes of stage D HF in patients with CHD, there is a need to integrate palliative care into the multidisciplinary care model for advanced HF in this population.

SUMMARY

HF is common in adults with CHD, United States, and it is the leading cause of death in this population. Adults with CHD presenting with stage D HF have a poor prognosis, and early recognition of signs of advanced HF, and referral for advanced therapies for HF offer the best survival as compared with other therapies. The indications for advanced therapies for HF outlined in this article should serve as a guide for clinicians to determine the optimal time for referral. Palliative care should be part of the multidisciplinary care model for HF in patients with CHD.

CLINICS CARE POINTS

- Early diagnosis and treatment heart failure (HF) is important in in adults with congenital heart disease (CHD).
- All adults with CHD should have a trial of guideline-directed medical therapy for HF.
- Early diagnosis of advanced HF and referral for advanced therapies for HF offer the best survival.

FUNDING

Dr A.C. Egbe is supported by National Heart, Lung, and Blood Institute (NHLBI), United States grants (R01 HL158517, R01 HL160761, and R01 HL162830).

DISCLOSURE

None.

REFERENCES

1. Egbe A, Uppu S, Stroustrup A, et al. Incidences and sociodemographics of specific congenital heart diseases in the United States of America: an evaluation of hospital discharge diagnoses. Pediatr Cardiol 2014;35:975–82.
2. Egbe A, Uppu S, Lee S, et al. Changing prevalence of severe congenital heart disease: a population-based study. Pediatr Cardiol 2014;35:1232–8.
3. Egbe A, Uppu S, Lee S, et al. Temporal variation of birth prevalence of congenital heart disease in the United States. Congenit Heart Dis 2015;10:43–50.
4. Diller GP, Arvanitaki A, Opotowsky AR, et al. Lifespan Perspective on Congenital Heart Disease Research: JACC State-of-the-Art Review. J Am Coll Cardiol 2021;77:2219–35.
5. Diller GP, Kempny A, Alonso-Gonzalez R, et al. Survival Prospects and Circumstances of Death in Contemporary Adult Congenital Heart Disease Patients Under Follow-Up at a Large Tertiary Centre. Circulation 2015;132:2118–25.
6. Tutarel O, Kempny A, Alonso-Gonzalez R, et al. Congenital heart disease beyond the age of 60: emergence of a new population with high resource utilization, high morbidity, and high mortality. Eur Heart J 2014;35:725–32.
7. Marelli AJ, Mackie AS, Ionescu-Ittu R, et al. Congenital heart disease in the general population: changing prevalence and age distribution. Circulation 2007;115:163–72.
8. Marelli AJ, Ionescu-Ittu R, Mackie AS, et al. Lifetime prevalence of congenital heart disease in the general population from 2000 to 2010. Circulation 2014;130:749–56.
9. Gilboa SM, Devine OJ, Kucik JE, et al. Congenital Heart Defects in the United States Estimating the Magnitude of the Affected Population in 2010. Circulation 2016;134:101–+.
10. Gilboa SM, Salemi JL, Nembhard WN, et al. Mortality resulting from congenital heart disease among children and adults in the United States, 1999 to 2006. Circulation 2010;122:2254–63.
11. Egbe AC, Miranda WR, Jain CC, et al. Prognostic Value of the Anatomic-Physiologic Classification in Adults With Congenital Heart Disease. Circulation Heart failure 2023;e010404.

12. Egbe AC, Miranda WR, Jain CC, et al. Temporal Changes in Clinical Characteristics and Outcomes of Adults With Congenital Heart Disease. Am Heart J 2023;264:1–9.

13. Engelings CC, Helm PC, Abdul-Khaliq H, et al. Cause of death in adults with congenital heart disease - An analysis of the German National Register for Congenital Heart Defects. Int J Cardiol 2016;211:31–6.

14. Verheugt CL, Uiterwaal CS, van der Velde ET, et al. Mortality in adult congenital heart disease. Eur Heart J 2010;31:1220–9.

15. McKee PA, Castelli WP, McNamara PM, et al. The natural history of congestive heart failure: the Framingham study. N Engl J Med 1971;285:1441–6.

16. Authors/Task Force M, McDonagh TA, Metra M, et al. 2021 ESC Guidelines for the diagnosis and treatment of acute and chronic heart failure: Developed by the Task Force for the diagnosis and treatment of acute and chronic heart failure of the European Society of Cardiology (ESC). With the special contribution of the Heart Failure Association (HFA) of the ESC. Eur J Heart Fail 2022;24:4–131.

17. Heidenreich PA, Bozkurt B, Aguilar D, et al. 2022 AHA/ACC/HFSA Guideline for the Management of Heart Failure: A Report of the American College of Cardiology/American Heart Association Joint Committee on Clinical Practice Guidelines. J Am Coll Cardiol 2022;79:e263–421.

18. Crespo-Leiro MG, Metra M, Lund LH, et al. Advanced heart failure: a position statement of the Heart Failure Association of the European Society of Cardiology. Eur J Heart Fail 2018;20:1505–35.

19. Egbe A, Miranda W, Connolly H, et al. Haemodynamic determinants of improved aerobic capacity after tricuspid valve surgery in Ebstein anomaly. Heart 2021;107:1138–44.

20. Egbe AC, Bonnichsen C, Reddy YNV, et al. Pathophysiologic and Prognostic Implications of Right Atrial Hypertension in Adults With Tetralogy of Fallot. J Am Heart Assoc 2019;8:e014148.

21. Egbe AC, Connolly HM, Miranda WR, et al. Hemodynamics of Fontan Failure: The Role of Pulmonary Vascular Disease. Circulation Heart failure 2017;10.

22. Egbe AC, Miranda WR, Connolly HM, et al. Coarctation of aorta is associated with left ventricular stiffness, left atrial dysfunction and pulmonary hypertension. Am Heart J 2021;241:50–8.

23. Egbe AC, Miranda WR, Anderson JH, et al. Prognostic Value of Left Ventricular Global Longitudinal Strain in Patients With Congenital Heart Disease. Circulation Cardiovascular imaging 2022;15:e014865.

24. Egbe AC, Miranda WR, Anderson JH, et al. Hemodynamic and Clinical Implications of Impaired Pulmonary Vascular Reserve in the Fontan Circulation. J Am Coll Cardiol 2020;76:2755–63.

25. Egbe AC, Younis A, Miranda WR, et al. Determinants and Prognostic Implications of Left Atrial Reverse Remodeling After Coarctation of Aorta Repair in Adults. Eur Heart J Cardiovasc Imaging 2023; jead203. https://doi.org/10.1093/ehjci/jead203.

26. Egbe AC, Miranda WR, Jain CC, et al. Prognostic Implications of Progressive Systemic Ventricular Dysfunction in Congenitally Corrected Transposition of Great Arteries. JACC Cardiovascular imaging 2022;15:566–74.

27. Egbe AC, Miranda WR, Connolly HM. Role of Echocardiography for Assessment of Cardiac Remodeling in Congenitally Corrected Transposition of Great Arteries. Circulation Cardiovascular imaging 2022;15:e013477.

28. Bokma JP, Geva T, Sleeper LA, et al. A propensity score-adjusted analysis of clinical outcomes after pulmonary valve replacement in tetralogy of Fallot. Heart 2018;104:738–44.

29. Geva T, Mulder B, Gauvreau K, et al. Preoperative Predictors of Death and Sustained Ventricular Tachycardia After Pulmonary Valve Replacement in Patients With Repaired Tetralogy of Fallot Enrolled in the INDICATOR Cohort. Circulation 2018;138:2106–15.

30. Lee MGY, Babu-Narayan SV, Kempny A, et al. Long-term mortality and cardiovascular burden for adult survivors of coarctation of the aorta. Heart 2019;105:1190–6.

31. Diller GP, Radojevic J, Kempny A, et al. Systemic right ventricular longitudinal strain is reduced in adults with transposition of the great arteries, relates to subpulmonary ventricular function, and predicts adverse clinical outcome. Am Heart J 2012;163:859–66.

32. Egbe AC, Miranda WR, Jain CC, et al. Prognostic Value of Cardiac Remodeling Staging in Adults With Repaired Coarctation of Aorta. JACC Cardiovascular imaging 2023;16:864–5.

33. Egbe AC, Miranda WR, Pellikka PA, et al. Prevalence and Prognostic Implications of Left Ventricular Systolic Dysfunction in Adults With Congenital Heart Disease. J Am Coll Cardiol 2022;79:1356–65.

34. Agarwal A, Dudley CW, Nah G, et al. Clinical Outcomes During Admissions for Heart Failure Among Adults With Congenital Heart Disease. J Am Heart Assoc 2019;8:e012595.

35. Zomer AC, Vaartjes I, van der Velde ET, et al. Heart failure admissions in adults with congenital heart disease; risk factors and prognosis. Int J Cardiol 2013;168:2487–93.

36. Stout KK, Daniels CJ, Aboulhosn JA, et al. 2018 AHA/ACC Guideline for the Management of Adults With Congenital Heart Disease: A Report of the American College of Cardiology/American Heart Association Task Force on Clinical Practice Guidelines. J Am Coll Cardiol 2019;73:e81–192.

37. Egbe AC, Miranda WR, Jain CC, et al. Incidence and Outcomes of Advanced Heart Failure in Adults With Congenital Heart Disease. Circulation Heart failure 2022;15:e009675.

38. Benedict CR, Johnstone DE, Weiner DH, et al. Relation of neurohumoral activation to clinical variables

and degree of ventricular dysfunction: a report from the Registry of Studies of Left Ventricular Dysfunction. SOLVD Investigators. J Am Coll Cardiol 1994; 23:1410–20.

39. Dunlay SM, Roger VL, Killian JM, et al. Advanced Heart Failure Epidemiology and Outcomes: A Population-Based Study. JACC Heart Fail 2021;9: 722–32.

40. Wang F, Liu A, Brophy JM, et al. Determinants of Survival in Older Adults With Congenital Heart Disease Newly Hospitalized for Heart Failure. Circulation Heart failure 2020;13:e006490.

41. Egbe AC, Adigun R, Anand V, et al. Left Ventricular Systolic Dysfunction and Cardiovascular Outcomes in Tetralogy of Fallot: Systematic Review and Meta-analysis. Can J Cardiol 2019;35:1784–90.

42. Egbe AC, Miranda WR, Ammash NM, et al. Atrial Fibrillation Therapy and Heart Failure Hospitalization in Adults With Tetralogy of Fallot. JACC Clin Electrophysiol 2019;5:618–25.

43. Egbe AC, Miranda WR, Jain CC, Connolly HM. Right Heart Dysfunction in Adults With Coarctation of Aorta: Prevalence and Prognostic Implications. Circ Cardiovasc Imaging 2021;14(12):1100–8.

44. Egbe AC, Miranda WR, Dearani J, et al. Left Ventricular Global Longitudinal Strain Is Superior to Ejection Fraction for Prognostication in Ebstein Anomaly. JACC Cardiovascular imaging 2021;14: 1668–9.

45. Egbe AC, Miranda WR, Dearani JA, et al. Hemodynamics and Clinical Implications of Occult Left Ventricular Dysfunction in Adults Undergoing Ebstein Anomaly Repair. Circulation Cardiovascular imaging 2021;14:e011739.

46. Andi K, Abozied O, Miranda WR, et al. Clinical benefits of angiotensin receptor-Neprilysin inhibitor in adults with congenital heart disease. Int J Cardiol 2023;387:131152.

47. Baumgartner H, De Backer J. The ESC Clinical Practice Guidelines for the Management of Adult Congenital Heart Disease 2020. Eur Heart J 2020; 41:4153–4.

48. Kempny A, Dimopoulos K, Uebing A, et al. Reference values for exercise limitations among adults with congenital heart disease. Relation to activities of daily life–single centre experience and review of published data. Eur Heart J 2012;33:1386–96.

49. Egbe AC, Connolly HM, Khan AR, et al. Outcomes in adult Fontan patients with atrial tachyarrhythmias. Am Heart J 2017;186:12–20.

50. Egbe AC, Connolly HM, McLeod CJ, et al. Thrombotic and Embolic Complications Associated With Atrial Arrhythmia After Fontan Operation: Role of Prophylactic Therapy. J Am Coll Cardiol 2016;68: 1312–9.

51. Egbe AC, Miranda WR, Anderson JH, et al. Determinants and Prognostic Implications of Hepatorenal Dysfunction in Adults With Congenital Heart Disease. Can J Cardiol 2022;38:1742–50.

52. Adams ED, Jackson NJ, Young T, et al. Prognostic utility of MELD-XI in adult congenital heart disease patients undergoing cardiac transplantation. Clin Transplant 2018;32:e13257.

53. Assenza GE, Graham DA, Landzberg MJ, et al. MELD-XI score and cardiac mortality or transplantation in patients after Fontan surgery. Heart 2013;99: 491–6.

54. Dimopoulos K, Diller GP, Koltsida E, et al. Prevalence, predictors, and prognostic value of renal dysfunction in adults with congenital heart disease. Circulation 2008;117:2320–8.

55. Egbe AC, Miranda WR, Jain CC, et al. Improvement in hepatic and renal function following isolated heart transplant in adults with congenital heart disease. Int J Cardiol 2022;364:44–9.

56. Egbe A, Miranda WR, Connolly HM, et al. Temporal changes in liver stiffness after Fontan operation: Results of serial magnetic resonance elastography. Int J Cardiol 2018;258:299–304.

57. Lindsay I, Johnson J, Everitt MD, et al. Impact of liver disease after the fontan operation. Am J Cardiol 2015;115:249–52.

58. Pundi K, Pundi KN, Kamath PS, et al. Liver Disease in Patients After the Fontan Operation. Am J Cardiol 2016;117:456–60.

59. Wu FM, Kogon B, Earing MG, et al. Landzberg MJ and Alliance for Adult Research in Congenital Cardiology I. Liver health in adults with Fontan circulation: A multicenter cross-sectional study. J Thorac Cardiovasc Surg 2017;153:656–64.

60. Egbe AC, Poterucha JT, Warnes CA, et al. Hepatocellular Carcinoma After Fontan Operation: Multicenter Case Series. Circulation 2018;138:746–8.

61. Bryant R 3rd, Rizwan R, Zafar F, et al. Contemporary Outcomes of Combined Heart-Liver Transplant in Patients With Congenital Heart Disease. Transplantation 2018;102:e67–73.

62. John AS, Johnson JA, Khan M, et al. Clinical outcomes and improved survival in patients with protein-losing enteropathy after the Fontan operation. J Am Coll Cardiol 2014;64:54–62.

63. John AS, Phillips SD, Driscoll DJ, et al. The use of octreotide to successfully treat protein-losing enteropathy following the Fontan operation. Congenit Heart Dis 2011;6:653–6.

64. Cedars A, Vanderpluym C, Koehl D, et al. An Interagency Registry for Mechanically Assisted Circulatory Support (INTERMACS) analysis of hospitalization, functional status, and mortality after mechanical circulatory support in adults with congenital heart disease. J Heart Lung Transplant 2018;37:619–30.

Special Considerations for Mechanical Circulatory Support or Device Therapy in Adult Congenital Heart Disease Heart Failure

Rafael Alonso-Gonzalez, MD, MSc, FESC[a],*, Guillermo Agorrody, MD[a]

KEYWORDS

- Heart failure • Mechanical circulatory support • Ventricular assist device • Fontan
- Systemic right ventricle

KEY POINTS

- Advanced heart failure is the leading cause of death in the adult congenital heart disease (ACHD) population.
- Heart transplant remains the treatment of choice in ACHD patients with end-stage heart failure.
- ACHD patients with biventricular circulation supported with ventricular assist devices (VADs) have similar survival to patients with acquired heart failure.
- Patients with Fontan circulatory failure and impaired systolic function benefit from VADs.
- Careful planning is essential for a good outcome and to prevent complications.

INTRODUCTION

Advances in the surgical and medical management of patients with complex congenital heart disease (CHD) have led to almost 90% of CHD patients reaching adulthood. Many of these patients will develop complications over time, such as arrhythmias, valvular or ventricular dysfunction, and ultimately heart failure. While heart failure is the leading cause of death in adult CHD (ACHD) patients after the fifth decade of life,[1,2] there is no evidence of the survival benefit of guideline-directed medical therapy (GDMT) in this population, particularly in patients with systemic right ventricle or univentricular physiology. Although the number of ACHD patients receiving a heart transplant has increased over time,[3] ACHD patients are listed at lower priority, have longer waitlist times, and are more likely to be delisted due to clinical decompensation or die while on the waiting list.[4] Mechanical circulatory support (MCS) is currently the standard of care strategy in acquired heart disease to restore systemic perfusion and allow cardiac recovery in patients with cardiogenic shock and is increasingly used as a bridge to transplant or as a destination therapy in patients with refractory heart failure. Despite recent data suggesting that MCS may be effective in reducing mortality in ACHD patients,[5,6] their use in this cohort is limited. This article will discuss the current evidence of MCS in ACHD patients and its potential challenges.

[a] Toronto ACHD Program, Division of Cardiology, Department of Medicine, Peter Munk Cardiac Centre, Toronto General Hospital, University Health Network, University of Toronto, 585 University Avenue, 5N-525, Toronto, Ontario, M5G 2N2, Canada
* Corresponding author.
E-mail address: rafa.alonso.g@gmail.com

Heart Failure Clin 20 (2024) 155–165
https://doi.org/10.1016/j.hfc.2023.12.003
1551-7136/24/© 2023 Elsevier Inc. All rights reserved.

HEART FAILURE AND ADVANCED THERAPIES IN CONGENITAL HEART DISEASE

Heart failure is the leading cause of death in the ACHD population after the fifth decade of life and one of the most common causes of hospitalization. Although the risk of developing heart failure is 2-fold to 3-fold higher in patients with complex CHD, patients with simple CHD have a 6.5% cumulative incidence of heart failure before the age of 40 years.[7] A recent study using the US National Inpatient Sample showed almost 8-fold increase in ACHD heart failure hospitalizations over a 10-year period with higher mortality amongst ACHD patients compared with those with acquired disease.[8] The heterogenous anatomy and physiology of ACHD patients makes the diagnosis and management of heart failure challenging in this population. While patients with simple lesions may present with similar signs and symptoms as acquired heart disease patients, atypical symptoms such as fatigue, inability to work, increased cyanosis, or diarrhea are the norm in complex CHD patients.

Although neurohormonal activation plays a role in ACHD heart failure, there are limited data to support the use of GDMT in patients with complex CHD; hence, initiation of medical therapy should not delay consideration of advanced therapies in this population. In addition, in ACHD patients with preload-dependent circulation, such as those with Fontan circulation, the use of medications that reduce afterload medication might lead to a reduction in cardiac output. It is, therefore, essential that there is a robust understanding of the underlying physiology of each individual CHD patient prior to starting GDMT.

The exact timing for referring ACHD patients for assessment for advanced heart failure therapies is yet to be defined. ACHD patients have a long-standing adaptation to their limitations. This leads to an under appreciation of the signs of deterioration. Atypical symptoms can also be missed if not followed by trained ACHD providers. In our group experience, following these patients in a dedicated ACHD heart failure clinic run by ACHD providers with training in heart failure provides better patient care and timely access to advance heart failure therapies in these patients.

ACHD patients may not be candidates for transplant for multiple reasons including complex anatomy, multiorgan dysfunction, high allosensitization, pulmonary hypertension, malignancy, obesity, social contraindications, or simply patient choice,[9] and in this setting, MCS may be considered. The use of MCS has increased exponentially in acquired heart disease patients and to a certain extent also in ACHD heart failure patients.[6] However, several anatomic and physiologic challenges make candidacy for MCS more challenging in the ACHD population.[10]

MECHANICAL CIRCULATORY SUPPORT IN ADULT CONGENITAL HEART DISEASE

A variety of devices are currently available for temporary or long-term hemodynamic support (**Fig. 1**). Depending on the mechanism of action, these devices can be classified as volume displacement, centrifugal, or axial flow pumps. Temporary circulatory support devices include, intra-aortic balloon pump, Impella devices, Tandem Heart, Centrimag, Rotaflow, and extracorporeal membrane oxygenation (ECMO). Long-term circulatory support devices are divided into intracorporeal ventricular assist devices (VADs; INCOR or Heartmate 3), paracorporeal (EXCOR), or total artificial heart (Syncardia TAH).[11]

Temporary Mechanical Circulatory Support in Adult Congenital Heart Disease

Temporary MCS can be used in ACHD patients as a bridge to recovery, a bridge to decision, a bridge to durable MCS, and, less commonly, a bridge to transplant. It is also used in high-risk patients during cardiac interventions, such as complex ablations. However, most of the evidence regarding the benefit of temporary circulatory support in ACHD comes from case reports or case series.[12–15] Comprehensive assessment of the peripheral vascular system and cardiac anatomy, with special attention to previous interventions that might have modified anatomic venous return (ie, bidirectional cavopulmonary anastomosis) or ventricular outflow (Damus-Kaye-Stansel procedure), is imperative when choosing the appropriate cannulation site.

Impella in adult congenital heart disease

The Impella devices (Abiomed, Danvers, MA, USA) are a series of nonpulsatile micro-axial flow pumps that can provide hemodynamic support up to 5 L/min. Currently there are 3 different devices based on the level of left ventricular support: Impella 2.5 (2.5 L/min, 12 Fr system), Impella cardiac power (CP) (3.5 L/min, 14 Fr system), and Impella 5.5 (5.0 L/min, 21 Fr system). The Impella 2.5 and CP can be placed percutaneously, whereas the Impella 5.5 requires a surgical cutdown with the device being delivered through a Dacron side graft on the axillary or femoral artery.[11]

Over the last few years, there have been several case reports and case series reporting the experience with Impella in patients with ACHD. Recently, Broda and colleagues[12] reported their experience

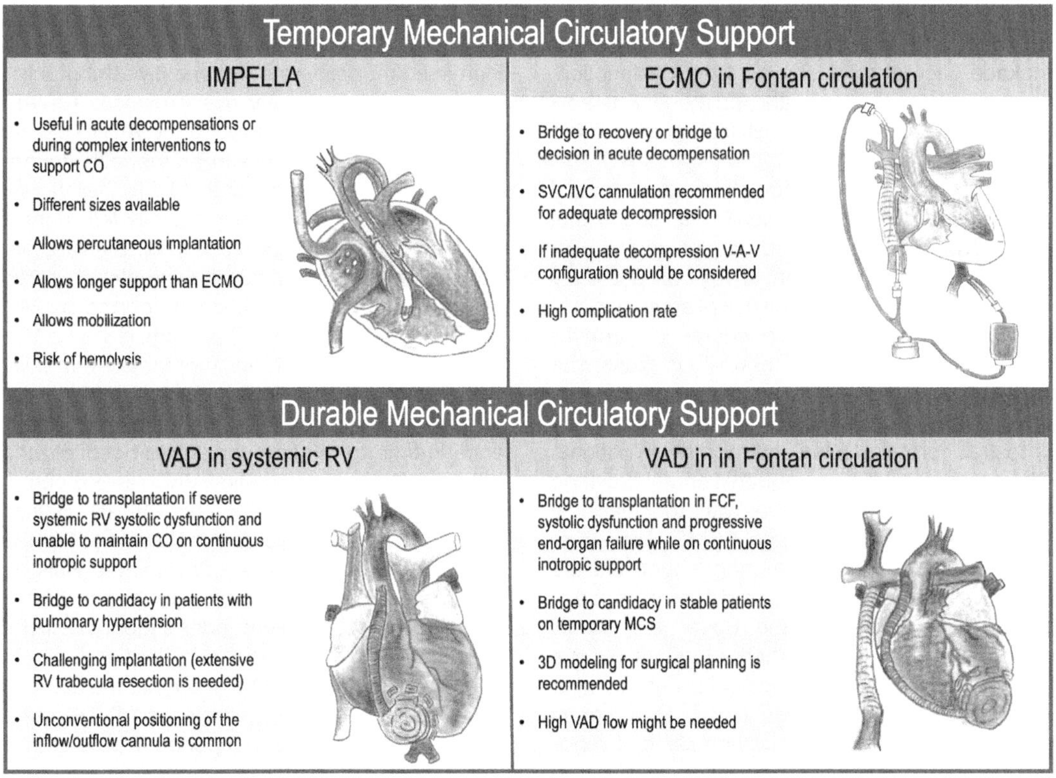

Fig. 1. Temporary and durable mechanical circulatory suppor in ACHD patients. CO, cardiac output; ECMO, extracorporeal membrane oxygenation; FCF, Fontan circulation failure; IVC, inferior vena cava; MCS, mechanical circulatory support; RV, right ventricle; SVC, superior vena cava; VAD, ventricular assist device; V-A-V, veno-arterial-venous.

in 6 patients (3 Fontan circulation; 2 biventricular circulation with systemic left ventricle; and 1 biventricular circulation with systemic right ventricle) who received either Impella CP, Impella 5.0, or Impella 5.5 (Abiomed Inc, Danvers, MA, USA) support. Four devices (57%) were placed in patients with acute decompensated heart failure and 3 devices (43%) were placed in patients with periprocedural hemodynamic compromise. The median time of support was 20 days (interquartile range (IQR) 3–44) and all 6 patients survived to hospital discharge. In 4 (67%) patients, the Impella was used as a bridge to recovery whereas bridge to durable MCS was the indication in the remaining 2 (33%). One patient developed severe hemolysis but otherwise there were no significant complications.

Choosing the correct device size and the appropriate cannulation site is essential. While an Impella CP might be appealing due to its size and percutaneous implantation, it may provide limited support requiring high-power settings which increase the risk of hemolysis whereas the Impella 5.5 with medium-power settings will provide adequate support with a much lower risk of hemolysis.[16] When compared to ECMO, Impella devices allow longer

support, up to ~5 weeks, have fewer complications, and achieve effective cardiac unloading.[16] In addition, if implanted via the axillary artery, they enable early mobilization and rehabilitation, helping the patient's recovery.

Extracorporeal membrane oxygenation in adult congenital heart disease

ECMO is a support modality used as a bridge to recovery or decision in the setting of acute decompensation, providing support for combined cardiopulmonary failure or in the setting of refractory cardiopulmonary arrest. In the postoperative setting, common indications for the use of ECMO in CHD patients include failure to wean from cardiopulmonary bypass, refractory low cardiac output syndrome, hemodynamically unstable arrhythmias, or extracorporeal cardiopulmonary resuscitation.[17]

Most of the ECMO data in ACHD are in the setting of postcardiotomy, with limited data in nonsurgical indications. Regardless of the indication, ACHD patients needing ECMO have a high risk of in-hospital mortality (between 57%[18] and 61%[13]), a higher rate of complications,[19] and longer hospital stay than non-ACHD patients.[19] Female gender, weight over 100 kg, delayed cannulation, neuromuscular blockade, acute renal injury, liver dysfunction, neurologic complications, and pulmonary hemorrhage have been reported as risk factors associated with increased mortality.[18,19]

Patients with Fontan circulation need special consideration. More specifically, a successful ECMO course with a Fontan patient begins with appropriate patient selection. While ECMO is likely to help Fontan patients at high risk of acute decompensation secondary to procedures or arrhythmias, it is likely to increase mortality in those with long-standing Fontan circulatory failure and end-organ dysfunction such as renal dysfunction, cirrhosis, or protein-losing enteropathy. In patients with Fontan circulation, adequate venous drainage might be difficult to achieve with the classical configuration of venous-arterial ECMO. Therefore, cannulation of the cavopulmonary shunt and the femoral vein should be considered if there is suboptimal decompression of the upper and lower venous compartments.[17] When adequate venous drainage is achieved, the systemic output must be fully supported with ECMO flow.[17] However, in the setting of incomplete decompression, a veno-arterial-venous configuration might be considered. This allows return of oxygenated blood into the Fontan circuit to promote flow through the circuit and return to the systemic ventricle. In addition to the benefit of stasis prevention, this will also ensure that the upper part of the body receives oxygenated blood.[17] If ECMO is placed in patients with Fontan circulation, it should be for a short period of time, and if recovery is not achieved, a more durable form of MCS should be considered.

Durable Mechanical Circulatory Support in Adult Congenital Heart Disease

Advances in durable MCS, especially with the development of left VADs (LVADs), have completely revolutionized the management of advanced heart failure. More than 2000 LVADs are annually implanted in the United States, almost half of them as a destination therapy.[20] However, data from 2015 indicated that only 0.8% of the Interagency Registry for Mechanically Assisted Circulatory Support (INTERMACS) was implanted in ACHD patients.[21] Reasons for this disparity between ACHD and non-ACHD patients most commonly include the anatomic and physiologic challenges, but probably the most limiting factor is the lack of data supporting the benefit and safety of these devices in the ACHD population.[22] The INTERMACS registry documented 126 ACHD patients with a VAD implanted between June 2006

and December 2015. ACHD patients had higher morbidity and mortality (**Fig. 2**A). However, the increased mortality rate was mostly attributable to patients on biventricular assist devices (BiVADs) or TAH (see **Fig. 2**C).[21] Importantly, ACHD patients with an LVAD showed similar mortality to non-ACHD patients independently of whether the systemic ventricle was morphologically left, right, or univentricular (see **Figs. 2**B and **3**). Similarly, in a competing outcomes analysis, a greater proportion of ACHD patients died while supported by MCS compared with non-ACHD patients (28% vs 19%; $P = .08$), primarily in the first months post-implant.[5] Interestingly, among patients with LVADs, this difference was not significant.[5,21] There was no difference in time to the first unplanned hospitalization after discharge or to the first VAD-related complication. Both ACHD and non-ACHD patients showed similar improvement in New York Heart Association functional class and 6-minute walk distance after the VAD implant. Age greater than 50 and BiVAD or TAH were independent predictors of mortality in ACHD patients in the first 5 months after MCS. Non-group O blood type, the presence of an implantable defibrillator, and INTERMACS patient profile 1 were independent predictors of mortality 6 months after implantation.[5] Morphology of the systemic ventricle, left, right, or univentricular, was not predictor of outcome.

In 2018, the United Network for Organ Sharing adult heart transplant allocation criteria changed from the previous 3-tier listing system to a 6-tier system to reduce waitlist mortality in very sick patients.[23] The new system favors ACHD patients with single ventricle requiring VAD support who are listed as status 2 under the new system. But there is still a selection bias against complex CHD patients with biventricular circulation and stable on VAD support. These patients get listed at the same status as any other CHD patient. However, in a cohort of 894 ACHD patients listed for transplant, those with VAD support at the time of listing (n = 91) had a higher waitlist mortality (38% vs 17%; $P<.01$).[24] Interestingly, there was no difference in 1-year post-transplant mortality between VAD versus non-VAD at the time of transplant (15% vs 17%; $P = .66$).[24] ECMO use was associated with significantly higher mortality (**Fig. 4**) with no significant difference. Body mass index less than 20 kg/m^2, bilirubin greater than 2 mg/dL, creatinine greater than 2 mg/dL, and ECMO at transplant were independent predictors of early post-transplant mortality.[24] This study highlights that ACHD patients supported by VAD do not have worse prognosis after transplant and should encourage ACHD heart failure providers to consider VAD in these patients as a bridge to heart transplantation when indicated.

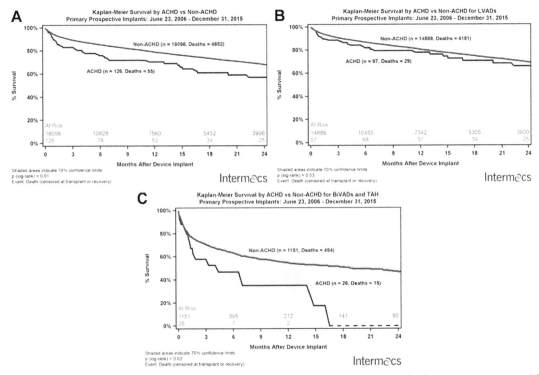

Fig. 2. (*A*) Kaplan-Meier survival after MCS implantation for all ACHD compared with all non-ACHD patients. (*B*) Kaplan-Meier survival after LVAD implantation for all ACHD compared with all non-ACHD patients. (*C*) Kaplan-Meier survival after BiVAD and TAH implantation for all ACHD compared with all non-ACHD patients. ACHD, adult congenital heart disease; BiVAD, biventricular assist device; LVAD, left ventricular assists devices; MCS, mechanical circulatory support; TAH, total artificial heart. (Reproduced with permission from VanderPluym CJ et al.[21])

General considerations

Durable VAD implantation should be considered in selected ACHD patients with favourable anatomy and poor quality of life or poor medium-term prognosis. In this population, it is important to understand the mechanism of failure prior to VAD implantation because the underlying physiology will play a role in their candidacy for MCS. Reversible causes of heart failure, significant comorbidities, or other life-limiting illnesses need to be excluded before VAD implantation.[25]

Durable VAD support in ACHD patients can be used as a bridge to transplantation, a bridge to candidacy, or as a destination therapy. While waitlist survival is better in ACHD patients with non-VAD support,[24] VAD should be considered as a bridge to transplantation in patients that are unable to maintain adequate cardiac output and end-organ perfusion with continuous inotropic support. In these patients, VAD may improve survival to transplantation. Pulmonary hypertension precluding heart transplantation is common in ACHD patients making these patients good candidates for VAD support as a bridge to candidacy.[26]

In patients with systemic right ventricle, implantation of a durable VAD has shown to reduce transpulmonary gradient with most patients becoming transplant eligible within the first-year postimplantation.[16] Although VAD implantation as a destination therapy is one of the most common indications of VAD implantation in acquired heart disease,[25] it remains a marginal indication in ACHD patients.[21] Recovery of the left ventricular function after VAD implantation is unusual in ACHD patients but it can be seen in about 5% of patients some acquired heart disease patients, with some of them having the device explanted at 5 years. Regardless of the initial VAD indication, it is important to have a clear strategy at the time of implantation and manage the patient expectations accordingly, with special consideration to the psychological burden of living with a VAD. As previously stated by Modica and colleagues[27], "*LVAD makes you independent from heart failure but does not allow an independent life.*" Involvement of the palliative care team and having discussions on advanced directive and end-of-life care are also imperative.

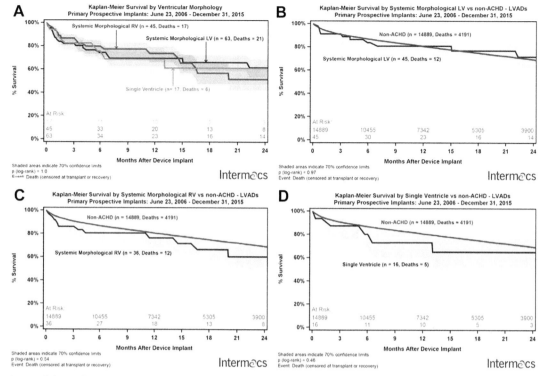

Fig. 3. (*A*) Kaplan-Meier survival after MCS implantation for all ACHD patients divided by ventricular morphology. (*B*) Kaplan-Meier survival after LVAD implantation for patients with a systemic morphologic left ventricle. (*C*) Kaplan-Meier survival after LVAD implantation for patients with a systemic morphologic right ventricle. (*D*) Kaplan-Meier survival after LVAD implantation for patients with a single ventricle. ACHD, adult congenital heart disease; LV, left ventricle; LVAD, left ventricular assists devices; MCS, mechanical circulatory support; RV, right ventricle. (Reproduced with permission from VanderPluym CJ et al.[21])

VAD implantation in ACHD can be challenging. All durable VADs are designed to be implanted in patients with levocardia and a left-sided systemic left ventricle. Detailed surgical planning is needed in most of the patients, especially in those with complex anatomy, such as situs inversus, dextrocardia, systemic right ventricle, or univentricular heart. Preimplantation 3D and virtual reality studies are encouraged to decide the type of device and the best implantation site.[9,28] The optimal pump

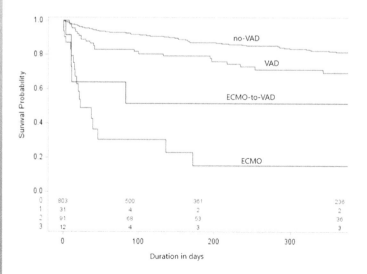

Fig. 4. Waitlist survival in adult congenital heart disease patients by mechanical circulatory support. ECMO, extracorporeal membrane oxygenation; VAD, ventricular assist device. (Reproduced with permission from Das BB et al.[24])

location will depend on the ventricular arrangement and mediastinal topology. Using intraoperative transoesophageal and intraoperative epicardial echocardiography is recommended to guide the implantation and confirm unobstructed inflow cannula position.[16,29] In patients with systemic right ventricle, diaphragmatic or anterolateral right ventricular free wall implantation of the inflow cannula is common with special attention to avoid the tricuspid valve sub-valvar apparatus and not to abut the septum.[16] Aggressive trabeculation resection is also performed in these patients.[9] The outflow cannula will be positioned leftward or right ward, depending on the anatomy of the patient and will be anastomosed to the ascending aorta, although alternative locations may be considered such as the innominate artery[29]

Anticoagulation is necessary for all VADs to decrease thromboembolic complications. Anticoagulation strategies vary by device, institutional practices, and individual patient factors such as previous surgeries, end-organ function, or associated comorbidities.[30] For example, Fontan patients with protein-losing enteropathy or liver disease may be at higher risk of both bleeding and/or thrombus formation due to loss of antithrombotic factors[30]

Durable ventricular assist devices in systemic right ventricle

Although there are several CHDs where the right ventricle supports the systemic circulation, we will focus this section on the 2 conditions with biventricular circulation and a morphologically right ventricle in a subaortic position. These are patients with congenitally corrected transposition of the great arteries and patients with dextro-transposition of the great arteries (d-TGA) after Mustard or Senning repair. In this setting, the right ventricle supports the systemic circulation and most of the patients will develop moderate to severely impaired right ventricular systolic function by the forth decade of life.[31,32] In this population, the course of the disease is particularly rapid after the onset of heart failure which is associated with a significantly high risk of sudden death.[33] Patients with systemic right ventricle are also at risk of developing severe pulmonary hypertension, most of them due to increased end-diastolic pressure[26] resistant to medical therapy that will be a contraindication to heart transplantation. GDMT has not been shown to improve survival in these patients, and its initiation should not delay the consideration for advanced therapies.

Over the last years, several groups have reported their experience with VADs in patients with systemic right ventricle. Most of these publications report small single-center series. Recently, a study included 27 patients with systemic right ventricle.[16] Most of the patients were d-TGA after Mustard or Senning repair (20 [74%]) and bridge to candidacy was the indication in 19 patients (70%) whereas bridge to transplant was the indication in 5 (19%). In the remaining 3 patients (11%), the indication for VAD was destination therapy. The majority of the patients (25 [93%]) were alive at discharge and 76% of discharge survivors became transplant eligible. Out of 19 patients where the VAD was implanted as bridge to candidacy, in 16 patients the indication was elevated transpulmonary gradient. Out of these 16 patients, most of them (13 [81%]) became transplant eligible.

The unusual position and anatomy of the right ventricle makes the implantation of the inflow and outflow cannulas challenging. Although apical implantation can be achieved in some cases, the diaphragmatic surface of the systemic right ventricle is the most common location for the inflow cannula.[16,29] In addition, the device might need to be placed back-to-front, closer to the midline, or through the right chest, to avoid damage of the liver or chamber compression upon closure of the chest.[34] Aggressive resection of right ventricle trabeculations is essential to avoid obstruction of the inflow cannula, although this is less common with the third generation VADs, mainly with the Heart-Mate 3 that has a shorter inflow cannula. Concomitant surgeries at the time of VAD implantation such as baffle revision or tricuspid valve replacement might need to be considered.

Durable ventricular assist devices in single ventricle

Survival of patients with Fontan circulation has improved significantly over the last 50 years, with 80% of patients alive at the age of 40.[35] As they age, Fontan patients are at risk for developing arrhythmia, thromboembolic events, protein-losing enteropathy, liver and renal dysfunction, and ultimately heart failure, all of which increase their risk of mortality. The current estimated 5-year mortality rate of a 40-year-old Fontan patient is approximately 20%, equivalent to a 75-year-old non-ACHD patient.[1,35] Given the increasing number of patients with Fontan circulation worldwide, more than 1000 Fontan operations are performed per year only in the United States,[36] and the number of patients with Fontan circulatory failure, the need of advanced heart failure therapies will grow in the coming years.

Over the last 5 to 10 years, there has been increasing evidence showing the benefit of VAD support in pediatric patients with Fontan circulatory failure and ventricular systolic dysfunction.[37,38]

However, the experience in ACHD patients remains limited to case series or individual case reports.[9,21,39,40] The indication for VAD support in patients with Fontan circulation is not yet established, but VAD support might be considered as a bridge to transplant in patients with Fontan circulatory failure, systolic dysfunction, and progressive end-organ failure while on intravenous inotropes, or as a bridge to candidacy in stable patients on temporary MCS. With the development of new durable devices with fewer complications, some groups are currently offering VAD support as a destination therapy to patients with Fontan circulatory failure who are not ideal transplant candidates or who do not wish to proceed to transplant.[36]

Exhaustive assessment prior VAD implantation is paramount to understand the mechanism of Fontan circulatory failure and to identify potential treatable causes that will not respond to VAD therapy. Patients with Fontan circulatory failure due to single ventricle dysfunction benefit the most from VAD therapy, while patients with normal systolic function and normal end-diastolic pressure, severe diastolic dysfunction, or inefficient Fontan flow are less likely to respond.[36,38] Planning should be started earlier, before patients develop severe complications such as irreversible liver dysfunction, hepatocellular carcinoma, or severe protein-losing enteropathy.[36,41] Evaluation of veno-venous and arteriovenous collaterals is important to understand postoperative cyanosis and how much the collateral flow contributes to the systemic circulation. Virtual implantation may be especially useful in Fontan patients to decide where to implant the inflow and outflow cannulas and to assess the best location for the pump within the thorax.[36] Absolute contraindications to VAD placement include irreversible and nontreatable end-organ damage, especially severe neurologic injury, and active infection.[36,42] Leaving a fenestration at the time of implantation to secure VAD flow and minimize the risk of suction events in situations where passive pulmonary blood flow may be reduced is recommended by some groups.[36] Early extubation and ambulation are strongly recommended. It is important to mention that given that aortopulmonary collateral flow often accounts for 15% to 30% of aortic flow in Fontan patients, VAD flow should run higher than normal in these patients to fully decompress the single ventricle.[36]

Two large registries of single ventricle MCS support in pediatric and adolescent patients, including intracorporeal and paracorporeal devices, temporary MCS, and left a right VAD, have been recently published with most of the patients alive on support or successfully transplanted, suggesting that VAD support can be an realistic option in these patients.[36,37] In a recent report, 8 adults and 1 pediatric patient with Fontan circulatory failure were treated with an implantable centrifugal-flow durable VADs. The median age at the time of implant was 24 years (IQR, 19–35 years) and the most common indication was bridge to candidacy (67%), followed by bridge to transplant (33%). HeartMate 3 was the most used device. Out of the 9 patients, 5 patients (55.6%) were successfully discharged home, 2 patients (22.2%) were transplanted before discharge, and 2 patients died from multiorgan failure (22.2%). Out of the 5 patients discharged home, 4 were successfully transplanted, most of them within the first-year post-discharge, and 1 remained on the device at the time of the publication. The median time of VAD support was 65 days (IQR, 27–360 days), with the longest duration being 1105 days. Of the 7 patients that survived, all maintained good renal function or had an improvement in renal function after placement of the VAD. Similarly, 5 patients had a decrease or no change in total bilirubin levels. The most common complications were driveline or systemic infections followed by hematological disorders, with only 1 patient having a hemorrhagic stroke.[41]

Future directions

While the experience with VAD support in patients with Fontan circulation is growing and the results are encouraging, this does not address all forms of Fontan circulatory failure. Patients with normal systolic function and severe diastolic function, the most common mode of failure in the ACHD population, and patients with limited pulmonary blood flow, such as those with elevated PVR, do not benefit from this therapy. New strategies are needed to support the failing Fontan circulation due to these mechanisms. There have been several pediatric cases of successful implantation of the TAH (SynCardia, Tucson, Arizona, USA) in patients with Fontan circulation,[37] with at least 1 patient being successfully bridged to transplant.[43] Unfortunately, the complexity of the surgical placement and the small number of centers with adequate experience in the management of these patients have resulted in high in-hospital mortality.[22] Biventricular VAD support with 2 continuous flow VADs is another option. However, the current available devices make this challenging. In a first-in-man study of the new Berlin Heart EXCOR Venous Cannula (EXCOR Venous Cannula, Berlin Heart GmbH, Berlin, Germany), a cannula was specifically developed to support pediatric patients with univentricular physiology by facilitating implantation of the EXCOR device into the Fontan pathway in combination with a systemic MCS.[44]

Over the last 10 years there has been growing interest in developing implantable cavopulmonary assist device that will simultaneously reduce systemic venous pressure and increase pulmonary arterial pressure, improving preload and cardiac output, in a univentricular Fontan circulation on a long-term basis.[45] However, these devices remain under development.

SUMMARY

Advanced heart failure is the leading cause of death in the ACHD population. While heart transplantation remains the treatment of choice in those with end-stage disease, ACHD patients have longer waiting time and higher mortality and delisting rates while awaiting transplant. MCS has rapidly evolved over the last 10 years, and it is now widely used in patients with acquired heart disease. ACHD patients with biventricular circulation supported with VAD have similar survival and improvement in quality of life to patients with acquired heart failure. There is also increasing evidence suggesting that patients with Fontan circulatory failure and impaired systolic function benefit from VAD. Therefore, MCS should be offered to ACHD patients in a timely fashion.

CLINICS CARE POINTS

- The risk of developing heart failure in patients with CHD increases over time and becomes the leading cause of death after the fifth decade of life.

- While patients with simple CHD lesions may present with similar heart failure signs and symptoms than patients with acquired heart disease, atypical symptoms, such as fatigue, inability to work or cyanosis, are common in patients with complex CHD.

- Treatment with GDMT should be considered in patients with simple CHD, however, there is scanty evidence for those with complex CHD, especially in patients with systemic right ventricle or single ventricle physiology and its initiation should not delay the consideration for advanced therapies.

- Temporary MCS can be used in ACHD patients as a bridge to recovery, a bridge to decision, a bridge to durable MCS, and, less commonly, a bridge to transplant. It can also be used in high-risk patients during cardiac interventions, such as complex ablations.

- Regardless of the indication, ACHD patients needing ECMO have a high risk of in-hospital mortality, higher rate of complications, and longer hospital stay than non-ACHD patients.

- When compared to ECMO, Impella devices in ACHD patient allow longer support, up to ~5 weeks, have fewer complications, and achieve effective cardiac unloading.

- Durable VAD implantation should be considered in selected ACHD patients with favourable anatomy and poor quality of life or poor medium-term prognosis and can be used as a bridge to transplantation, a bridge to candidacy, or as a destination therapy.

DISCLOSURE

None of the authors have any disclosures.

REFERENCES

1. Diller GP, Kempny A, Alonso-Gonzalez R, et al. Survival Prospects and Circumstances of Death in Contemporary Adult Congenital Heart Disease Patients Under Follow-Up at a Large Tertiary Centre. Circulation 2015;132(22):2118–25.
2. Oliver JM, Gallego P, Gonzalez AE, et al. Impact of age and sex on survival and causes of death in adults with congenital heart disease. Int J Cardiol 2017;245:119–24.
3. Karamlou T, Hirsch J, Welke K, et al. A United Network for Organ Sharing analysis of heart transplantation in adults with congenital heart disease: outcomes and factors associated with mortality and retransplantation. J Thorac Cardiovasc Surg 2010;140(1):161–8.
4. Alshawabkeh LI, Hu N, Carter KD, et al. Wait-List Outcomes for Adults With Congenital Heart Disease Listed for Heart Transplantation in the U.S. J Am Coll Cardiol 2016;68(9):908–17.
5. Cedars A, Vanderpluym C, Koehl D, et al. An Interagency Registry for Mechanically Assisted Circulatory Support (INTERMACS) analysis of hospitalization, functional status, and mortality after mechanical circulatory support in adults with congenital heart disease. J Heart Lung Transplant 2018;37(5):619–30.
6. Gelow JM, Song HK, Weiss JB, et al. Organ allocation in adults with congenital heart disease listed for heart transplant: impact of ventricular assist devices. J Heart Lung Transplant 2013;32(11):1059–64.
7. Gilljam T, Mandalenakis Z, Dellborg M, et al. Development of heart failure in young patients with congenital heart disease: a nation-wide cohort study. Open Heart 2019;6(1):e000858.
8. Burstein DS, Rossano JW, Griffis H, et al. Greater admissions, mortality and cost of heart failure in adults with congenital heart disease. Heart 2021; 107(10):807–13.
9. Perry T, Lorts A, Morales DLS, et al. Chronic Ventricular Assist Device Support in Adult Congenital Heart

Disease Patients: A Children's Hospital Perspective. ASAIO J 2021;67(12):e216–20.

10. Givertz MM, DeFilippis EM, Landzberg MJ, et al. Advanced Heart Failure Therapies for Adults With Congenital Heart Disease: JACC State-of-the-Art Review. J Am Coll Cardiol 2019;74(18):2295–312.

11. Atti V, Narayanan MA, Patel B, et al. A Comprehensive Review of Mechanical Circulatory Support Devices. Heart Int 2022;16(1):37–48.

12. Broda CR, Frankel WC, Nair AP, et al. Continuous-Flow Ventricular Assist Device Support in Adult Congenital Heart Disease: A 15-Year, Multicenter Experience of Temporary and Durable Support. ASAIO J 2023;69(5):429–37.

13. Dolgner SJ, Keeshan BC, Burke CR, et al. Outcomes of Adults with Congenital Heart Disease Supported with Extracorporeal Life Support After Cardiac Surgery. ASAIO J 2020;66(10):1096–104.

14. Maybauer MO, Vohra A, O'Keeffe NJ, et al. Extracorporeal membrane oxygenation in adult congenital heart disease: a case series and literature review. Crit Care Resusc 2017;19(Suppl 1):15–20.

15. Morray BH, Dimas VV, Lim S, et al. Circulatory support using the impella device in fontan patients with systemic ventricular dysfunction: A multicenter experience. Catheter Cardiovasc Interv 2017;90(1):118–23.

16. Roche SL, Crossland DS, Adachi I, et al. Mechanical Circulatory Support for the Failing Sub-Aortic Right Ventricle in Adults. Semin Thorac Cardiovasc Surg Pediatr Card Surg Annu 2021;24:2–9.

17. Bacon MK, Gray SB, Schwartz SM, et al. Extracorporeal Membrane Oxygenation (ECMO) Support in Special Patient Populations-The Bidirectional Glenn and Fontan Circulations. Front Pediatr 2018;6:299.

18. O'Neil E, Riedl R, Rycus P, et al. Extracorporeal membrane oxygenation support for adult congenital heart disease. J Am Coll Cardiol 2022;79(9_Supplement):570.

19. Kops SA, White SC, Klewer SE, et al. ECMO in adults with congenital heart disease - Analysis of a national discharge database. Int J Cardiol Congenit Heart Dis 2022;8:100366.

20. Kormos RL, Cowger J, Pagani FD, et al. The Society of Thoracic Surgeons Intermacs Database Annual Report: Evolving Indications, Outcomes, and Scientific Partnerships. Ann Thorac Surg 2019;107(2):341–53.

21. VanderPluym CJ, Cedars A, Eghtesady P, et al. Outcomes following implantation of mechanical circulatory support in adults with congenital heart disease: An analysis of the Interagency Registry for Mechanically Assisted Circulatory Support (INTERMACS). J Heart Lung Transplant 2018;37(1):89–99.

22. Monaco J, Khanna A, Khazanie P. Transplant and mechanical circulatory support in patients with adult congenital heart disease. Heart Fail Rev 2020;25(4):671–83.

23. Organ Procurement and Transplantation Network. Policy 6: allocation of hearts and heart-lungs. Richmond, VA: OPTN. 2018 (cited 2021 Aug 02). Available from: https://unos.org/news/the-new-adult-heart-allocation-policy-is-now-in-effect/. Accessed date 02 August 2021.

24. Das BB, Kogon B, Deshpande SR, et al. Contemporary outcomes of durable ventricular assist devices in adults with congenital heart disease as a bridge to heart transplantation. Artif Organs 2022;46(4):697–704.

25. Bhagra SK, Pettit S, Parameshwar J. Implantable left ventricular assist device: indications, eligibility and current outcomes. Heart 2022;108(3):233–41.

26. Van De Bruaene A, Toh N, Hickey EJ, et al. Pulmonary hypertension in patients with a subaortic right ventricle: prevalence, impact and management. Heart 2019;105(19):1471–8.

27. Modica M, Ferratini M, Torri A, et al. Quality of life and emotional distress early after left ventricular assist device implant: a mixed-method study. Artif Organs 2015;39(3):220–7.

28. Farooqi KM, Saeed O, Zaidi A, et al. 3D Printing to Guide Ventricular Assist Device Placement in Adults With Congenital Heart Disease and Heart Failure. JACC Heart Fail 2016;4(4):301–11.

29. Peng E, O'Sullivan JJ, Griselli M, et al. Durable ventricular assist device support for failing systemic morphologic right ventricle: early results. Ann Thorac Surg 2014;98(6):2122–9.

30. Santamaria RL, Jeewa A, Cedars A, et al. Mechanical Circulatory Support in Pediatric and Adult Congenital Heart Disease. Can J Cardiol 2020;36(2):223–33.

31. Roos-Hesselink JW, Meijboom FJ, Spitaels SE, et al. Decline in ventricular function and clinical condition after Mustard repair for transposition of the great arteries (a prospective study of 22-29 years). Eur Heart J 2004;25(14):1264–70.

32. Verheugt CL, Uiterwaal CS, van der Velde ET, et al. Mortality in adult congenital heart disease. Eur Heart J 2010;31(10):1220–9.

33. Kammeraad JA, van Deurzen CH, Sreeram N, et al. Predictors of sudden cardiac death after Mustard or Senning repair for transposition of the great arteries. J Am Coll Cardiol 2004;44(5):1095–102.

34. Haranal M, Luo S, Honjo O. Mechanical Circulatory Support for Patients With Adult Congenital Heart Disease. Circ J 2020;84(4):533–41.

35. Dennis M, Zannino D, du Plessis K, et al. Clinical Outcomes in Adolescents and Adults After the Fontan Procedure. J Am Coll Cardiol 2018;71(9):1009–17.

36. Villa CR, Lorts A, Morales DLS. Ventricular Assist Device Therapy in the Fontan Circulation. Semin

Thorac Cardiovasc Surg Pediatr Card Surg Annu 2021;24:19–25.

37. Bedzra EKS, Adachi I, Peng DM, et al. Systemic ventricular assist device support of the Fontan circulation yields promising outcomes: An analysis of The Society of Thoracic Surgeons Pedimacs and Intermacs Databases. J Thorac Cardiovasc Surg 2022; 164(2):353–64.

38. Cedars A, Kutty S, Danford D, et al. Systemic ventricular assist device support in Fontan patients: A report by ACTION. J Heart Lung Transplant 2021; 40(5):368–76.

39. Morales DL, Adachi I, Heinle JS, et al. A new era: use of an intracorporeal systemic ventricular assist device to support a patient with a failing Fontan circulation. J Thorac Cardiovasc Surg 2011;142(3): e138–40.

40. Woods RK, Ghanayem NS, Mitchell ME, et al. Mechanical Circulatory Support of the Fontan Patient. Semin Thorac Cardiovasc Surg Pediatr Card Surg Annu 2017;20:20–7.

41. Fahnhorst SE, Brandewie K, Perry T, et al. Single Center Experience With Durable Continuous Flow Single Ventricle Assist Device: A Viable Option in Fontan Circulatory Failure. ASAIO J 2023. https://doi.org/10.1097/MAT.0000000000001986.

42. Reid CS, Kaiser HA, Heinisch PP, et al. Ventricular assist device for Fontan: who, when and why? Curr Opin Anaesthesiol 2022;35(1):12–7.

43. Rossano JW, Goldberg DJ, Fuller S, et al. Successful use of the total artificial heart in the failing Fontan circulation. Ann Thorac Surg 2014;97(4):1438–40.

44. Karner B, Urganci E, Schlein J, et al. First-in-man use of the EXCOR Venous Cannula for combined cavopulmonary and systemic ventricular support in Fontan circulation failure. J Heart Lung Transplant 2022;41(10):1533–6.

45. Rodefeld MD, Marsden A, Figliola R, et al. Cavopulmonary assist: Long-term reversal of the Fontan paradox. J Thorac Cardiovasc Surg 2019;158(6): 1627–36.

Adults with Congenital Heart Disease and Transplant
Challenges, Opportunities, and Policy

Nicole Herrick, MD[a], Marcus Urey, MD[a], Laith Alshawabkeh, MD, MSCI[b],*

KEYWORDS

- ACHD heart failure • ACHD transplant • ACHD listing criteria

KEY POINTS

- Adults with congenital heart disease (ACHD) are increasingly developing heart failure; they are a heterogenous population and often present with atypical heart failure symptoms.
- ACHD patients undergoing evaluation for advanced heart failure therapies should undergo a more robust pretransplant, multidisciplinary assessment.
- The 1-year posttransplant mortality remains higher for ACHD patients, though we believe a robust pretransplant assessment and close monitoring for expected complications postoperatively can mitigate this risk.

CHALLENGES
A Heterogeneous Population with Atypical Heart Failure Symptoms

As the growing population of adults congenital heart disease (ACHD) enters adulthood, heart failure remains the primary cause of death.[1] The etiology of heart failure in ACHD is heterogeneous, driven by residual anatomic/structural abnormalities, arrhythmias, and ventricular dysfunction.[2–5] This is further compounded by traditional risk factors for acquired heart disease such as coronary disease, hypertension, diabetes, renal dysfunction, and obesity. Patients with ACHD often do not present with the typical symptomatic decline associated with heart failure; thus, it can be challenging to identify and determine the appropriate time to initiate an advanced therapies evaluation.

Most patients with ACHD do not progress linearly through the stages of heart failure. All ACHD patients by definition have structural abnormalities (stage B) and most have had prior heart failure symptoms; thus, most of the patients with ACHD will be in at least stage C heart failure. The New York Heart Association (NYHA) class can also be misleading as many have had poor exertional capacity their whole life and by the time they present with worsening symptoms they are severely decompensated.[5,6]

Classic physical examination findings including jugular venous distention and peripheral edema are also often unreliable in ACHD patients, particularly for those with the Fontan circulation. Natriuretic peptide levels are chronically elevated in patients with ACHD,[7,8] the degree of baseline elevation varies with the underlying anatomy, and there remain insufficient data to establish lesion-specific normal values. However, an acute increase above the individual's baseline correlates with worsening symptoms and may be helpful in monitoring for decompensation.[9]

Objective testing with cardiopulmonary exercise testing is frequently used to track disease course.

[a] Division of Cardiovascular Medicine, Department of Medicine, University of Calilfornia San Francisco, 505 Parnassus Avenue, San Francisco, CA 94143, USA; [b] Adult Congenital Heart Disease Program, Division of Cardiovascular Medicine, Department of Medicine, University of California, San Diego, 9452 Med Center Drive, ACTRI-3E, Mail 7411, La Jolla, CA 92037, USA
* Corresponding author.
E-mail address: lalsh@health.ucsd.edu

Heart Failure Clin 20 (2024) 167–174
https://doi.org/10.1016/j.hfc.2023.12.009

Table 1
Adults with congenital heart disease lesion-specific risk factors for the development of heart failure

Underlying Substrate	Disease	Mechanism
Systemic RV	D-loop TGA with atrial switch L-loop TGA HLHS	Chronic pressure and volume overload - > myocardial disarray, fibrosis, ischemia
Arrhythmia	TOF Eisenmenger syndrome Single ventricle, Fontan Systemic RV	Myofibroblast activation - > fibrosis - > arrhythmia
Cyanosis	Single-ventricle physiology Unrepaired congenital heart disease	Cyanosis promotes collateral formation - > AV collaterals leads to over circulation, volume overload, pulmonary vascular disease
Left to right shunting	VSD, ASD, PAPVR	Left- or right-sided volume overload
Valvular abnormalities	Congenital vs acquired	Volume or pressure overload

Abbreviations: ASD, atrial septal defect; AV, aortic valve; PAPVR, partial anomalous pulmonary venous return; TOF, tetralogy of fallot; VSD, ventricular septal defect.

It is generally accepted that a peak oxygen consumption (V_{O_2}) less than 50% of age predicted is characteristic of heart failure,[10] though there are no established lesion-specific normal values. Exercise capacity is uniformly decreased in ACHD patients, even in the absence of symptoms[6]; thus, a change over time in the individual V_{O_2} max is most predictive of decline, rather than using an absolute cutoff or normal value.

Given the difficulty using clinical symptoms to monitor for disease progression, those at highest risk should be followed more closely. **Table 1** outlines the lesion-specific risk factors for the development of heart failure.

One of the highest risk groups is those with a systemic right ventricle, including dextro-transposition of the great arteries (dTGA) who underwent an atrial switch, congenitally corrected TGA (or L-looped transposition of the great arteries [ITGA]), and hypoplastic left heart syndrome (HLHS).[2,11] The absence of the middle circular layer of myocardial fibers in the right ventricle (RV) may contribute to the inability to tolerate chronically elevated pressures leading to myocardial disarray, fibrosis, and ischemia.[2,11] In addition, the dilation and altered geometry of the failing RV predisposes to severe atrioventricular valve regurgitation in excess of what has been observed in those with a failing systemic left ventricle.[11]

The development of arrhythmias, particularly for those with tetralogy of Fallot, Eisenmenger syndrome, and the Fontan circulation, increases the risk of development of heart failure by two to threefold.[12] In patients with the Fontan circulation, atrial tachycardia is an independent predictor of death and hospital admission.[13] In addition, cyanosis and hypoxia promote the formation of collateral vessels, which over time can cause over circulation and contribute to volume overload and the development of pulmonary vascular disease.

Lapses in Care During the Transition to Adult Congenital Cardiology

The transition from pediatric to adult congenital cardiology is a high-risk time for lapses in care, which is associated with poor outcomes and increased overall mortality.[14] Lapses in care occur in 30% to 60% of patients with ACHD,[14] one study found that patients experiencing a lapse in care were more than twice as likely to need urgent or emergent intervention at the time of representation.[15] There is considerable effort underway to address the social determinants of health in ACHD patients, which invariably impacts clinical outcomes (**Fig. 1**).[16]

The Challenge with Sensitization

An additional risk factor for ACHD patients is their past exposure to human leukocyte antigen (HLA) antibody generating products and tissues. Multiple prior surgeries, exposure to blood products, pregnancy, and presence of synthetic homograft/allograft material all contribute to higher panel reactive antibody (PRA) levels observed in ACHD

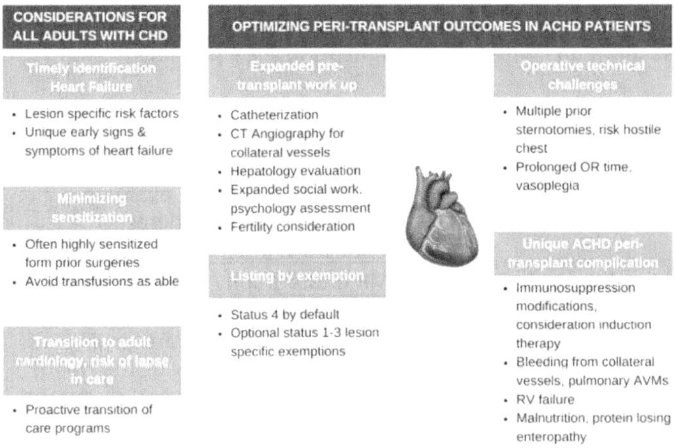

CONSIDERATIONS FOR ALL ADULTS WITH CHD

OPTIMIZING PERI-TRANSPLANT OUTCOMES IN ACHD PATIENTS

Timely identification Heart Failure
- Lesion specific risk factors
- Unique early signs & symptoms of heart failure

Minimizing sensitization
- Often highly sensitized form prior surgeries
- Avoid transfusions as able

Transition to adult cardiology, risk of lapse in care
- Proactive transition of care programs

Expanded pre-transplant work up
- Catheterization
- CT Angiography for collateral vessels
- Hepatology evaluation
- Expanded social work, psychology assessment
- Fertility consideration

Listing by exemption
- Status 4 by default
- Optional status 1-3 lesion specific exemptions

Operative technical challenges
- Multiple prior sternotomies, risk hostile chest
- Prolonged OR time, vasoplegia

Unique ACHD peri-transplant complication
- Immunosuppression modifications, consideration induction therapy
- Bleeding from collateral vessels, pulmonary AVMs
- RV failure
- Malnutrition, protein losing enteropathy

Fig. 1. Considerations and optimizing peritransplant outcomes in ACHD patients.

patients. PRA levels above 10% are considered significantly elevated, although routinely ACHD patients have PRAs well above 25%.[17] Higher PRA levels are associated with acute cellular rejection, early graft failure, as well as antibody-mediated rejection.[17] Although patients with ACHD are known to have higher PRA levels, the elevated PRA level alone does not fully explain the observed higher perioperative mortality posttransplantation.[18] This highlights the need to explore other factors, including operative complexity, bleeding risk, vasoplegia, and RV failure, which may be contributing to elevated early posttransplant mortality. In patients with protein-losing enteropathy and hypogammaglobinemia, PRA may be unreliable in assessing their true immunologic risk and rejection from an amnestic response when the immune system reconstitutes.

Operative and Technical Challenges

ACHD patients have altered anatomic and hemodynamic consequences of prior palliative surgeries in childhood. For example, patients with the Fontan circulation may require surgical reconstruction of their pulmonary arteries or systemic veins at the time of transplantation, adding to the procedural length and complexity.[2] Their unique circulation may alter the capacity of the liver or the kidney to withstand transplantation to a point where they may require liver transplantation or perioperative dialysis. Patients with a history of transposition of the great arteries palliated with an atrial switch operation may require systemic venous reconstruction at the time of transplantation. In our experience, many of such risks can be mitigated by multidisciplinary planning and careful investigation of "bystander" organ dysfunction.

OPPORTUNITIES

Opportunities: *In a carefully selected and thoroughly evaluated population, ACHD patients stand to gain more in the long-term from transplantation.*

The rate of heart transplantation in patients with ACHD is rising; as of 2021, patients with ACHD represent 3.3% of all transplants—roughly a 40% increase in the last 25 years.[2,19,20] The 1-year posttransplant survival is lower for ACHD compared with non-ACHD patients (85% vs 93%),[21] though those who survive the first year have significantly better 10-year posttransplant survival (49% vs 41%).[4] The improved long-term mortality has been attributed to younger age and fewer comorbid conditions in ACHD patients.[4]

Much of the differences in early mortality in our experience can be addressed by a robust pretransplant assessment, with careful patient selection and pretransplantation surgical planning. The transplant workup for ACHD patients is thorough and time-consuming. Listing patients while hospitalized for an acutely decompensated heart failure carries high risk for death before or after transplantation.[2,5,22,23]

The development of a multidisciplinary listing team is at the center of a robust pretransplant assessment. Team members should include adult congenital cardiology specialists, advanced heart failure/transplant subspecialists, adult cardiac transplant surgeons, pediatric cardiac transplant surgeons, psychologists, and social workers.

Table 2 summarizes the additional workup that should be considered for ACHD patients in addition to the standard pretransplant evaluation.

All ACHD patients with cyanosis should be formally evaluated for the development of collateral vessels and/or pulmonary arteriovenous malformations, and if present, should be intervened

Table 2
Supplemental pretransplant assessment for adults with congenital heart disease patients

Catheterization	Evaluate for collateral vessels, and evaluate pulmonary vascular resistance as appropriate
CT angiography of the chest and peripheral vasculature, consider 3D reconstruction to assist with surgical planning	Evaluate for collateral vessels, evaluate venous anatomy, and peripheral cannulation strategy
Hepatology referral	Consider MR elastography ± liver biopsy
Genetics, maternal fetal medicine referral	Delineate family planning strategies, consideration of pretransplant fertility preservation, counseling about the risk of transmission of congenital heart disease to offspring if this is pursued
Social work and cognitive assessment	In depth psychological assessment, depending on age consider standardized transition of care assessment. Executive functioning assessment

on preoperatively. This is typically done via coiling in the catheterization laboratory, though larger vessels may need to be surgically ligated at the time of transplant. Unrecognized and/or untreated collateral vessels greatly increase the intraoperative bleeding risk and may prolong circulatory arrest time. In addition, the increased venous return from unrepaired aortopulmonary collaterals is often not tolerated by the newly transplanted heart causing volume overload, complicating early postoperative recovery.

Experienced operators in congenital heart disease should perform the pretransplant hemodynamic assessment. A standard right heart catheterization is prone to inaccuracies for patients with ACHD. Owing to the presence of residual shunts, collateral vessels, and multiple sources of pulmonary blood flow, it can be challenging to accurately measure the true pulmonary vascular resistance. The combination of advanced imaging and appropriate catheterization allows the measurement of the pulmonary vascular resistance in most patients. As with many with ACHD, an individualized approach to each patient is encouraged rather than inflexible standardized hemodynamic cutoffs.

Patients with ACHD prone to chronic venous congestion should undergo a formal hepatology assessment. Certain anatomic lesions, especially those with the Fontan circulation and subpulmonic ventricular failure, are at the highest risk for hepatic fibrosis, though all ACHD patients born before 1990 should be screened for hepatitis C in the setting of childhood exposure to blood products. A liver biopsy is the gold standard for evaluating liver dysfunction, though MR elastography is increasingly used in lower risk patients. Partnering

with hepatologists with knowledge and skills in managing Fontan-associated liver disease is paramount because it requires specialized imaging and clinical approach to liver evaluation compared with other types of hepatic diseases.

It is also important to consider the technical surgical challenges of transplanting an ACHD patient. Regardless of the underlying anatomy, having undergone prior surgeries adds to the technical and operative challenges. This can significantly lengthen the surgical time, increasing the risk of vasoplegia and bleeding.[24] Patients often require peripheral cannulation to allow a safer chest reentry–preoperative evaluation of the peripheral venous and arterial tree is critical. An additional consideration is the need for pulmonary arterial reconstruction. Often if significant pulmonary artery or vein reconstruction is needed, a donor will only be accepted if they are not also donating the lungs, given the need to harvest more of the distal pulmonary vasculature than is standard. Some of these risks can be mitigated through robust surgical planning. Cardiac computed tomography (CT) with 3 dimensional (3D) reconstruction can assist with surgical planning and intraoperative efficiency. Overall, transplantation at centers with a higher volume of transplantation and those with an experienced adult congenital heart disease program led to better 30-day and 1-year survival posttransplantation.[25,26]

Patients with ACHD are significantly younger at the time of transplantation. Thus, family planning should be included in the transplant workup. This is particularly important for women, where it has been shown that pregnancy posttransplant, while feasible, has considerable risks to the fetus, the

Table 3
Peritransplant complications specific to patients with history of adults with congenital heart disease

RV failure	Dobutamine and milrinone as first line and can consider epinephrine
Prolonged OR time	Vasoplegia, and need for *early* hemodialysis
Collateral vessels • Common in patients with preoperative cyanosis • Increase circulatory arrest time, and volume overload posttransplant	Can be difficult to identify and missed even with robust preoperative evaluation. Consultation with the ACHD providers is paramount
Pulmonary AVMs • More common in patients with Fontan circulation • Persistent cyanosis posttransplant, and potentially volume overload	Addressing macro-AVMs if possible preoperatively; surveillance postoperatively for micro-AVMs
Malnutrition • Protein-losing enteropathy can persist for months posttransplantation	Robust nutritional assessment and support. Lymphatic intervention if feasible.
Immunosuppression • Consideration of induction therapy with maintenance steroids improved outcomes in some ACHD patients Many patients with Fontan circulation lack a thymus (excised during palliation surgery in childhood) and/or a functional spleen. Induction therapy is not routinely used in this population	Favor induction in highly sensitized patients, especially in those at risk for perioperative kidney failure. Monitor for bleeding, rATG can be associated with elevated bleeding risk.

Abbreviations: AVMs, arterial venous malformations; OR, operating room.

mother, and the transplanted heart.[4,27] Although transplant is no longer an absolute contraindication to pregnancy, it is recommended that women wait for at least 1-year posttransplantation and will need to consult closely with advanced heart failure and maternal–fetal medicine before conception to switch to a non-teratogenic immunosuppression regimen.[28,29] If they have experienced a significant rejection episode, it is strongly recommended that pregnancy is avoided entirely.[29,30] Men are also at risk for fertility issues posttransplantation. The highest risk is the development of hypogonadism and erectile dysfunction.[31] In young individuals of childbearing potential, it is important to discuss family planning and to set expectations for what may or may not be feasible in the posttransplant period. Thus, we recommend that all individuals with ACHD, regardless of gender, meet with a genetics counselor, fertility specialist, and maternal–fetal medicine as a part of the pretransplant assessment.

In addition to an expanded pretransplant assessment, an opportunity to improve the 1-year posttransplant mortality for ACHD patients is careful attention to potential postoperative hemodynamic complications unique to ACHD patients. The 30-day mortality is 17.4% for ACHD patients compared with 7.4% for non-ACHD patients.[2,22] **Table 3** outlines the common complications that should be proactively assessed in the peritransplant period.

The intricacies of the pretransplant evaluation and posttransplant care highlight the importance of being cared for at a center with ACHD subspecialists and a robust multidisciplinary team.

POLICY
Adults with Congenital Heart Disease Patients, as a Rule, Are an Exemption: How to Optimize Listing Priority?

In 2018, the United Network for Organ Sharing (UNOS) heart transplant listing guidelines were updated to the well-established status 1–7 system. With this updated listing criteria, patients with ACHD are, by default, listed as a status 4. Many ACHD patients are ineligible for much of the standard criteria to achieve higher listing status (mechanical circulatory support [MCS] devices, continuous pulmonary artery catheters). Thus, they need an additional exception for higher listing status. There are established prespecified exception rules for unique situations that could be used, especially in patients with the Fontan circulation. Successfully submitting this additional exception relies on the center's expertise and understanding with transplanting ACHD patients.[32] This highlights the importance of appropriately timing the referral to heart failure specialists. The ACTION network recently outlined Fontan-specific complications that should prompt a timely referral for transplant evaluation. Criteria included systemic ventricular dysfunction, Fontan pathway dysfunction, lymphatic dysfunction (presenting as protein-losing enteropathy or plastic bronchitis), and extracardiac dysfunction (including fontan associated liver disease [FALD] with synthetic dysfunction or hepatocellular carcinoma, chronic kidney disease stage 3 or higher, and hemoptysis).[33]

Overall, the 2018 policy change is considered to be beneficial for ACHD patients. There have now been multiple studies[34] that examined waitlist and transplant rates before and after the 2018 policy change showing the waitlist time decreased significantly (161 vs 38 days, $P < .001$) without any significant change in 1-year mortality.

Status 1 Exemptions	Single-ventricle physiology • With temporary or permanent MCS with dysfunction
Status 2 Exemptions	Single-ventricle physiology • Continuous inotropes (high dose or multiple mid-range doses), inotrope intolerance, *without* a requirement for continuous hemodynamic monitoring
Status 3 Exemptions	Single-ventricle physiology • With ACHD-specific complications including plastic bronchitis, protein-losing enteropathy, conduit thrombosis

What About Mechanical Circulatory Support Devices?

The updated 2018 UNOS guidelines emphasized the use of temporary MCS devices, automatically upgrading listing to status 2.[35] However, many ACHD patients are not candidates for MCS devices due to underlying anatomy (Fontan circulation, residual shunting, and so forth), risk of additional sensitization, and lack of robust evidence of its use in ACHD patients.[35] Often MCS is considered a last resort in ACHD patients. Unsurprisingly, outcomes in early observational studies have been poor.[23,36] However, more contemporary studies suggest that in carefully selected patients, outcomes are probably similar to non-ACHD patients.[37,38]

CLINICS CARE POINTS

- Adults with congenital heart disease have unique lesion specific risk factors and clinical presentation of heart failure that can delay advanced heart failure evaluation.
- Adults with congenital heart disease benefit from a robust multidisclipinary pre-transplant evaluation at a center with ACHD expertise.

DISCLOSURE

The authors have no relevant financial disclosures.

REFERENCES

1. Verheugt C, Uiterwaal C, van der Velde E, et al. Mortality in adult congenital heart disease. Eur Heart J 2010; 31(10). https://doi.org/10.1093/eurheartj/ehq032.
2. Bryant R, Morales D. Overview of adult congenital heart transplants. Ann Cardiothorac Surg 2018; 7(1). https://doi.org/10.21037/acs.2018.01.01.
3. Yap S, Harris L, Chauhan V, et al. Identifying high risk in adults with congenital heart disease and atrial arrhythmias. Am J Cardiol 2011;108(5). https://doi.org/10.1016/j.amjcard.2011.04.021.
4. Doumouras B, Alba A, Foroutan F, et al. Outcomes in adult congenital heart disease patients undergoing heart transplantation: a systematic review and meta-analysis. J Heart Lung Transplant 2016;35(11). https://doi.org/10.1016/j.healun.2016.06.003.
5. Alshawabkeh L, Opotowsky A. Burden of heart failure in adults with congenital heart disease. Curr Heart Fail Rep 2016;13(5). https://doi.org/10.1007/s11897-016-0301-0.
6. Diller G, Dimopoulos K, Okonko D, et al. Exercise intolerance in adult congenital heart disease: comparative severity, correlates, and prognostic implication. Circulation 2005;112(6). https://doi.org/10.1161/CIRCULATIONAHA.104.529800.
7. Norozi K, Wessel A, Alpers V, et al. Incidence and risk distribution of heart failure in adolescents and adults with congenital heart disease after cardiac surgery. Am J Cardiol 2006;97(8). https://doi.org/10.1016/j.amjcard.2005.10.065.
8. Eindhoven J, van den Bosch A, Ruys T, et al. N-terminal pro-B-type natriuretic peptide and its relationship with cardiac function in adults with congenital heart disease. J Am Coll Cardiol 2013;62(13). https://doi.org/10.1016/j.jacc.2013.07.019.
9. Miyamoto K, Takeuchi D, Inai K, et al. Prognostic value of multiple biomarkers for cardiovascular mortality in adult congenital heart disease: comparisons of single-/two-ventricle physiology, and systemic

morphologically right/left ventricles. Heart Ves 2016; 31(11). https://doi.org/10.1007/s00380-016-0807-0.

10. Kempny A, Dimopoulos K, Uebing A, et al. Reference values for exercise limitations among adults with congenital heart disease. Relation to activities of daily life–single centre experience and review of published data. Eur Heart J 2012;33(11). https://doi.org/10.1093/eurheartj/ehr461.

11. Menachem J, Schlendorf K, Mazurek J, et al. Advanced heart failure in adults with congenital heart disease. JACC Heart failure 2020;8(2). https://doi.org/10.1016/j.jchf.2019.08.012.

12. Miller J, Simpson K, Epstein D, et al. Improved survival after heart transplant for failed Fontan patients with preserved ventricular function. J Heart Lung Transplant 2016;35(7). https://doi.org/10.1016/j.healun.2016.02.005.

13. Giannakoulas G, Dimopoulos K, Yuksel S, et al. Atrial tachyarrhythmias late after Fontan operation are related to increase in mortality and hospitalization. Int J Cardiol 2012;157(2). https://doi.org/10.1016/j.ijcard.2010.12.049.

14. Gurvitz M, Valente A, Broberg C, et al. Prevalence and predictors of gaps in care among adult congenital heart disease patients: HEART-ACHD (The Health, Education, and Access Research Trial). J Am Coll Cardiol 2013;61(21). https://doi.org/10.1016/j.jacc.2013.02.048.

15. Yeung E, Kay J, Roosevelt G, et al. Lapse of care as a predictor for morbidity in adults with congenital heart disease. Int J Cardiol 2008;125(1). https://doi.org/10.1016/j.ijcard.2007.02.023.

16. John A, Jackson J, Moons P, et al. Advances in managing transition to adulthood for adolescents with congenital heart disease: a practical approach to transition program design: a scientific statement from the American heart association. J Am Heart Assoc 2022;11(7). https://doi.org/10.1161/JAHA.122.025278.

17. Kaufman B, Shaddy R. Immunologic considerations in heart transplantation for congenital heart disease. Curr Cardiol Rev 2011;7(2). https://doi.org/10.2174/157340311797484204.

18. Alshawabkeh L, Herrick N, Opotowsky A, et al. The role of sensitization in post-transplant outcomes in adults with congenital heart disease sensitization in adults with congenital heart disease. Int J Cardiol Congenit Heart Dise 2022;8.

19. Goldfarb SB, Levvey BJ, Edwards LB, et al. The registry of the international society for heart and lung transplantation: nineteenth pediatric lung and heart-lung transplantation report-2016; focus theme: primary diagnostic indications for transplant. J Heart Lung Transplant 2016;35(10):1196–205.

20. Kinsella A, Rao V, Fan C, et al. Post-transplant survival in adult congenital heart disease patients as compared to dilated and ischemic cardiomyopathy patients; an analysis of the thoracic ISHLT registry. Clin Transplant 2020;34(9). https://doi.org/10.1111/ctr.13985.

21. Dolgner S, Nguyen V, Krieger E, et al. Long-term adult congenital heart disease survival after heart transplantation: A restricted mean survival time analysis. J Heart Lung Transplant 2021;40(7). https://doi.org/10.1016/j.healun.2021.02.019.

22. MM G, EM D, MJ L, et al. Advanced heart failure therapies for adults with congenital heart disease: jacc state-of-the-art review. J Am Coll Cardiol 2019;74(18). https://doi.org/10.1016/j.jacc.2019.09.004.

23. Davies RR, Russo MJ, Yang J, et al. Listing and transplanting adults with congenital heart disease. Circulation 2011;123(7):759–67.

24. Lewis M, Ginns J, Schulze C, et al. Outcomes of adult patients with congenital heart disease after heart transplantation: impact of disease type, previous thoracic surgeries, and bystander organ dysfunction. J Card Fail 2016;22(7). https://doi.org/10.1016/j.cardfail.2015.09.002.

25. JN M, J L, K S, et al. Center volume and post-transplant survival among adults with congenital heart disease. J Heart Lung Transplant 2018;37(11). https://doi.org/10.1016/j.healun.2018.07.007.

26. VP N, SJ D, TF D, et al. Improved outcomes of heart transplantation in adults with congenital heart disease receiving regionalized care. J Am Coll Cardiol 2019; 74(23). https://doi.org/10.1016/j.jacc.2019.09.062.

27. Acuna S, Zaffar N, Dong S, et al. Pregnancy outcomes in women with cardiothoracic transplants: a systematic review and meta-analysis. J Heart Lung Transplant 2020;39(2):93–102.

28. Dagher O, Alami Laroussi N, Carrier M, et al. Pregnancy after heart transplantation: a well-thought-out decision? the Quebec provincial experience - a multi-centre cohort study. Transpl Int 2018. https://doi.org/10.1111/tri.13144.

29. Costanzo MR, Dipchand A, Starling R, et al. The international society of heart and lung transplantation guidelines for the care of heart transplant recipients. J Heart Lung Transplant 2010;29(8):914–56.

30. Durst JK, Rampersad RM. Pregnancy in women with solid-organ transplants: a review. Obstet Gynecol Surv 2015;70(6):408–18.

31. Thirumavalavan N, Scovell J, Link R, et al. Does solid organ transplantation affect male reproduction? European Urology Focus 2018;4(3). https://doi.org/10.1016/j.euf.2018.08.012.

32. Review Board (RB). Guidance for adult congenital heart disease (CHD) exception requests. USA: Organ Procurement and Transplantation Network (OPTN) Website Guidelines; 2017.

33. AM L, A C, CS A, et al. Considerations for advanced heart failure consultation in individuals with Fontan circulation: recommendations from action. Circulation Heart Failure 2023;16(2). https://doi.org/10.1161/CIRCHEARTFAILURE.122.010123.

34. Kainuma A, Ning Y, Kurlansky P, et al. Changes in waitlist and posttransplant outcomes in patients with adult congenital heart disease after the new heart transplant allocation system. Clin Transplant 2021;35(11). https://doi.org/10.1111/ctr.14458.

35. McMahon A, McNamara J, Griffin M. A review of heart transplantation for adults with congenital heart disease. J Cardiothorac Vasc Anesth 2021;35(3). https://doi.org/10.1053/j.jvca.2020.07.027.

36. Everitt M, Donaldson A, Stehlik J, et al. Would access to device therapies improve transplant outcomes for adults with congenital heart disease? Analysis of the United Network for Organ Sharing (UNOS). J Heart Lung Transplant 2011;30(4). https://doi.org/10.1016/j.healun.2010.09.008.

37. VanderPluym C, Cedars A, Eghtesady P, et al. Outcomes following implantation of mechanical circulatory support in adults with congenital heart disease: an analysis of the interagency registry for mechanically assisted circulatory support (INTERMACS). J Heart Lung Transplant 2018;37(1). https://doi.org/10.1016/j.healun.2017.03.005.

38. Rizwan R, Bryant R, Zafar F, et al. Inferior transplant outcomes of adolescents and young adults bridged with a ventricular assist device. ASAIO (American Society for Artificial Internal Organs : 1992) 2018;64(3). https://doi.org/10.1097/MAT.0000000000000685.

Arrhythmias in Adult Congenital Heart Disease Heart Failure

Anudeep K. Dodeja, MD[a], Shailendra Upadhyay, MD[b],*

KEYWORDS

- Adult congenital heart disease • Arrhythmia • Heart failure • Sudden cardiac arrest catheter ablation
- Pacemaker • Defibrillator

KEY POINTS

- Heart failure and arrhythmias represent 2 major causes of mortality and morbidity in adults with congenital heart disease.
- Arrhythmias and heart failure are interdependent, and one may exacerbate the other. Treatment of one also has a positive impact on the other.
- Management approaches need to be multifaceted, including pharmacotherapy, optimization of hemodynamic status with catheter based or surgical interventions, and specific management of arrhythmia with device or catheter ablation therapy

INTRODUCTION

Heart failure (HF) and arrhythmia represent 2 major contributors to mortality and morbidity in adult congenital heart disease (ACHD) population. Bradyarrhythmia and tachyarrhythmia are both common in ACHD patients. HF is the leading cause of morbidity and mortality in this unique growing population accounting for 17% to 42% of all ACHD deaths.[1–5]

Over 50% of patients with complex congenital heart disease (CHD) will develop atrial arrhythmias (AA) by the age of 65.[6,7] Arrhythmias increase the risk for HF and cardiac intervention by 2 to 3 times.[7] Atrial tachycardia is an independent predictor of death and hospitalization in patients with tetralogy of Fallot (TOF) and Fontan circulation.[8–10] Sudden cardiac death (SCD) is a leading cause of mortality in ACHD patients, which can occur in even otherwise stable ACHD patients in their third or fourth decade of life .[1,2,9] SCD is reported to occur between 7% and 44% among different ACHD

conditions.[11] In this article, the authors will review the interplay between HF and arrhythmia in different forms of ACHD and the management strategies.

ARRHYTHMIA AND HEART FAILURE: A PERNICIOUS COMBINATION IN ADULT CONGENITAL HEART DISEASE

Over the course of their lifetime, nearly half of ACHD patients will develop arrhythmias, and one-hird will experience systemic or pulmonary venous congestion.[12] ACHD patients may exhibit a pre-existing arrhythmia substrate, consequences of changes in hemodynamic burden, or impacts resulting from the type of surgical intervention (**Fig. 1**, **Table 1**).[13]

The intricate relationship between HF and arrhythmogenesis is becoming increasingly acknowledged.[14] Common risk factors for the development of arrhythmia and HF in ACHD comprise advancing age, the complexity of the underlying CHD, the quantity and nature of prior cardiac surgeries, and

[a] Division of Pediatric Cardiology, Department of Pediatrics, Connecticut Children's, University of Connecticut School of Medicine, 282 Washington Street, Hartford, CT 06106, USA; [b] Department of Pediatric Cardiology, Connecticut Children's, University of Connecticut School of Medicine, 282 Washington Street, Hartford, CT 06106, USA
* Corresponding author.
E-mail address: supadhyay@connecticutchildrens.org

Heart Failure Clin 20 (2024) 175–188
https://doi.org/10.1016/j.hfc.2023.12.004

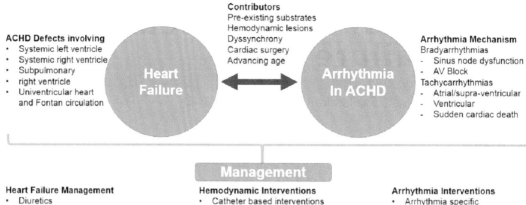

Fig. 1. The correlation between heart failure and arrhythmia in adults with congenital heart disease (ACHD). It also demonstrates the multifaceted management strategies targeted specifically at addressing arrhythmia, alleviating the hemodynamic burden, and implementing the failure-specific therapies.

acquired heart diseases.[15] As indicated in the table, numerous CHD conditions are inherently predisposed to causing bradyarrhythmias (such as sinus node dysfunction [SND] and AV block), tachyarrhythmias (including AA and supraventricular tachycardia), as well as conduction disturbances or bundle branch blocks. Tachyarrhythmias can potentially lead to tachycardia-mediated cardiomyopathy and subsequent ventricular dysfunction. Meanwhile, bradyarrhythmias, junctional rhythms, and heart block may contribute to HF by compromising cardiac output, stemming from excessively slow heart rates or the loss of atrioventricular synchrony. Patients presenting with profound bundle branch block or chronic pacing requirements might develop pacemaker or dyssynchrony-mediated ventricular dysfunction. Myocardial dysfunction could arise from previous cardiac surgeries, cardio-pulmonary bypass, valvular heart diseases, pericardial abnormalities, outflow obstruction, and volume/pressure loading of the ventricles. Additionally, interventions such as patches and baffles might induce myocardial remodeling, leading to chamber dilation, fibrosis, and altered myocardial refractory periods. Mechanical-electrical interactions could act as triggers for arrhythmia. The interplay between HF and arrhythmias can exacerbate each other; however, addressing one condition can offer benefit to the other. For example, the prompt management of tachyarrhythmias can aid in resolving tachycardia-mediated cardiomyopathy (**Fig. 2**).

AAs are notably the most prevalent arrhythmia within the ACHD population. Nevertheless,

ventricular arrhythmias stand out as the primary culprits behind SCD within this group. Statistics suggest that around 50% of individuals with ACHD in their 20s will experience an AA at some point during their lifespan.[6,13]

The prevalence of ventricular arrhythmias varies within the range 1% to 15% among different categories of ACHD. These occurrences are most commonly observed in patients with TOF (ranging from 10%-15%), followed by those with D-transposition of the great arteries (D-TGA) after atrial switch operations, which fall within a range of 7% to 9%.[13]

The authors will now explore the spectrum of ACHD conditions categorized according to the state of the systemic ventricle. These categories are outlined later. Disrupted mechanical and electrical interactions can contribute to either muscle dysfunction or arrhythmias (see **Fig. 2**).

Substrates and Mechanism of Arrhythmia and HF in ACHD: HF in ACHD may be categorized based on dysfunction involving various ventricular configurations, including the systemic left ventricle (LV), systemic right ventricle (RV), subpulmonary RV, or univentricular hearts.

Systemic Left Ventricle

Patients with CHD and biventricular physiology are susceptible to the development of LV dysfunction over time. This progression can arise due to residual lesions, such as valve disease, outflow tract obstruction, as well as factors like multiple cardiopulmonary bypass runs, abnormal coronary perfusion (either anatomic or due to injury during

Table 1
Summary of arrhythmia in different forms of ACHD

Congenital Heart Disease Diagnosis	Specific Diagnosis	Underlying or Acquired Sinus Node/AV Node/conduction System Abnormality	Pre-operative Arrhythmia Substrate	Post-Operative Arrhythmia Substrate
Systemic LV CHD	Left heart obstructive lesions • Aortic stenosis • Subaortic membrane Post Ross/Konno operation Coarctation of aorta	AV block (post Ross/Konno), in sub-aortic stenosis	VT	AFL AFib VT SCD
	Mitral Valve Disorders (stenosis or insufficiency)	AV block	AFL AFib	AFL AFib
	AV Canal defects and ventricular septal defect	AV block Twin AV Nodes	Twin node reentry	IART AFib
	Patent ductus arteriosus	-	-	VT
	ALCAPA	AV block	Ischemic LV	AFL IART AFib VT
Sub-pulmonary RV CHD	Atrial septal defect and PFO	SND (Sinus venosus type) after repair	AA	AFL IART AFib
	D-TGA, VSD, PS post Rastelli repair	AV block		AFL IART
	Ebstein anomaly	SND WPW syndrome/multiple accessory pathways	SVT (AVRT) AFL VT	AFL IART EAT VT SCD
	Double-chambered right ventricle and pulmonary stenosis	? SND	VT	? AFL
	Tetralogy of Fallot. post repair	SND	-	AFL/IART AFib NAFAT VT SCD
	Truncus arteriosus	AV block	-	AFL IART

(continued on next page)

Table 1
(continued)

Congenital Heart Disease Diagnosis	Specific Diagnosis	Underlying or Acquired Sinus Node/AV Node/conduction System Abnormality	Pre-operative Arrhythmia Substrate	Post-Operative Arrhythmia Substrate
Systemic RV CHD	D-TGA, post atrial switch operation	SND	-	AFL NAFAT AVNRT VT/VF
	Congenitally corrected TGA	SND AV block Accessory pathway	AVRT Twin node reentry	AVRT AFL
Univentricular hearts and Heterotaxy syndrome	Double inlet left ventricle	SND		IART AFL NAFAT
	Double outlet left right ventricle with hypoplastic left ventricle	SND Twin AV Nodes (S,L,L and I,L,L anatomy)	Twin node reentry	IART AFL NAFAT
	Hypoplastic left heart syndrome	SND		IART AFL NAFAT
	Heterotaxy syndrome	SND AV Block Twin AV nodes	Twin node reentry	IART AFL FAT
	Pulmonary atresia intact ventricular septum	SND		IART AFL NAFAT
	Tricuspid valve atresia	SND Left axis deviation		IART AFL NAFAT
	Unbalanced AV Canal	SND AV Block Twin AV nodes	Twin node reentry	IART AFL NAFAT

Abbreviations: AA, atrial arrhythmias; AFib, atrial fibrillation; AFL, atrial flutter; ALCAPA, anomalous origin of the left coronary artery from pulmonary artery; AVNRT, AV node reentry tachycardia; AVRT, atrio-ventricular reentry tachycardia; EAT, ectopic atrial tachycardia; IART, intra-atrial re-entrant tachycardia; NAFAT, non-automatic focal atrial tachycardia; PFO, patent foramen ovale; SCD, sudden cardiac death; SND, sinus node dysfunction; SVT, supraventricular tachycardia; TGA, transposition of the great arteries; VT, ventricular tachycardia.

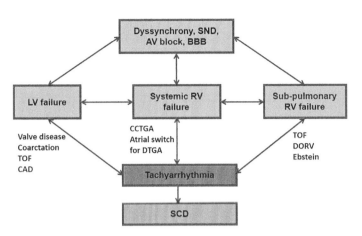

Fig. 2. The diagram illustrates the interaction between heart failure and arrhythmia in ACHD conditions involving systemic LV, systemic RV, and sub-pulmonary RV. BBB, bundle branch block; CAD, coronary artery disease; CCTGA, congenitally-corrected transposition of the great arteries; DORV, double outlet right ventricle; DTGA, D-transposition of the great arteries; SND, sinus node dysfunction; TOF, tetralogy of Fallot.

repair), arrhythmias, and associated cardiomyopathies. Notably, conditions like left ventricular noncompaction in Ebstein anomaly.

In tetralogy pf Fallot (TOF), the development of LV dysfunction frequently precedes and poses significant risk of death or hospitalization in patients with repaired TOF.[16]

LV systolic dysfunction is an independent predictor of death, aborted SCD, or sustained ventricular tachycardia. A systematic review and meta-analysis demonstrated a 30% increase in the risk of adverse cardiac events for every 5% decrease in left ventricular ejection fraction (LVEF), as well as a 3-fold increase in the risk of cardiovascular adverse events in patients with LVEF less than 40% compared with other patients.[17] While systolic dysfunction is a common cause of HF in CHD, diastolic HF is also prevalent, albeit difficult to quantify due to variable anatomy.[18] Systemic LV dysfunction is associated with an increased risk of atrial fibrillation.

Systemic Right Ventricle

There are 2 major groups representing systemic RV involvement. The first group comprises patients with D-TGA who have undergone an atrial switch operation (Mustard/Senning). The second group consists of patients with congenitally corrected transposition of the great arteries (CCTGA). Tricuspid valve insufficiency is often associated in both of these conditions and frequently precedes clinical HF.[19,20]

More than 50% of patients who have undergone Mustard/Senning repairs experience HF symptoms by the age of 40.[21] RV dysfunction and tricuspid regurgitation are risk factors for development of HF in this population along with a number of other long-term issues that contribute to symptomatic HF, including atrial and ventricular arrhythmias, heart block, and SND. Furthermore, these

patients also tend to have an extensive atrial scarring, leading to high incidence of AA.[22] Rapid atrioventricular (AV) conduction in the setting of an already compromised systemic RV can lead to induction of secondary ventricular tachycardia and SCD.[23,24]

Patients with CCTGA are at a high risk for heart block and/or SND, often necessitating chronic pacing. They are also vulnerable to accessory pathway–mediated tachycardia. Surprisingly, up to 24% of ACHD patients who require chronic pacing may eventually develop pacemaker-mediated cardiomyopathy.[20]

Subpulmonary Right Ventricle

The most common cause of sub-pulmonary RV failure in patients with CHD is secondary to pressure-loaded or volume-loaded RV. For example, this occurs in patients with TOF after repair, often accompanied by residual pulmonary stenosis and/or pulmonary regurgitation, as well as in patients with Ebstein anomaly and severe tricuspid regurgitation. In such cases, valve intervention should be considered to improve ventricular function. Maintenance of sinus rhythm and AV synchrony is particularly important in RV failure because atrial fibrillation and atrioventricular block may have profound hemodynamic effects.[25]

In presence of a tachyarrhythmia, the right atrial pressure increases.[26] In patients with intracardiac shunts at the atrial level, such as with atrial septal defects and Ebstein anomaly, this can lead to shunt reversal, cyanosis, and HF.

Univentricular Heart and Fontan Palliated Ventricles

Many forms of complex univentricular heart defects such as tricuspid atresia, hypoplastic left heart syndrome, double inlet left ventricle, unbalanced atrioventricular canal defect, certain forms of double outlet right ventricle, and pulmonary atresia with intact ventricular septum may require palliation with Fontan circulation. Fontan physiology represents a uniquely delicate state wherein there is no sub-pulmonary ventricle. The systemic veins (SVC and IVC) are directly connected to the pulmonary arteries, resulting in passive sub-pulmonary systemic venous flow, and the single ventricle (morphologically left or right ventricle) serves as the systemic ventricle.

The long-term effects of a Fontan circulation result in several complications including HF and arrhythmias.[27,28]

Adults with single ventricle physiology and Fontan palliation are at risk for developing SND and atrial tachyarrhythmias.[29] Approximately 90% of Fontan patients who experience heart failure–related deaths have concomitant AAs.[30]

The incidence of AAs following Fontan repairs varies by the type of surgery and duration of follow-up. The occurrence of late AAs has been reduced from 60% to less than 20% by surgical modifications. Late ventricular tachycardia is reported in 3% to 12% of patients. Aggressive efforts to eliminate tachycardia and enhance hemodynamics may lead to an improvement in clinical status.[31] The presence of ventricular arrhythmias in Fontan patients is highly associated with the need for transplantation or death.[32]

MANAGEMENT OF ARRHYTHMIA AND HEART FAILURE IN ADULT CONGENITAL HEART DISEASE

Management of HF and arrhythmia in ACHD necessitates a multifaceted approach. Treatment should be tailored to identify reversible causes, alleviate hemodynamic burden, and implement specific arrhythmia therapy. Acute HF resulting from primary arrhythmias (tachyarrhythmia or bradyarrhythmia) requires management with antiarrhythmic medications or device therapy. In contrast, HF in a failing Fontan circulation may mandate targeted interventions such as Fontan conversion or valve replacement, dependent on the underlying hemodynamic mechanism or addressing ventricular dyssynchrony.[12] (**Fig. 3**). Progressive HF upon addressing acute arrhythmia and hemodynamic burden requires guideline-directed medical therapy and evaluation of candidacy for advanced HF therapies including mechanical support and transplant.

MEDICAL MANAGEMENT/PHARMACOLOGIC THERAPY

Medications used for the management of HF can also yield positive effects on suppressing arrhythmia. Beta blockers (such as metoprolol succinate, and carvedilol) used for managing HF management have been shown to provide beneficial effects in reducing ventricular arrhythmias and the occurrence of SCD.[33,34] Sacubitril/valsartan may reduce the arrhythmic burden in patients with non-permanent atrial fibrillation (AF) and decrease the subclinical atrial tachycardia/atrial fibrillation (AT/AF) episodes in patients with no prior history of AF, but it may not have the same effects in patients with permanent AF.[35]

Pharmacologic therapy for arrhythmia and HF presents challenges in the ACHD population due to concurrent tachycardia-bradycardia syndrome arising from prevalent SND. Rate and rhythm control of atrial arrhythmias constitute the foundation of anti-arrhythmic drug therapy. AV nodal blocking agents including class II-beta blockers and class IV-calcium channel blockers are employed for rate control. However, calcium channel blockers carry the potential to induce HF due to their negative inotropic effects. Both class II and IV agents entail the risk of exacerbating SND and AV block.

Class I agents such as intravenous procainamide or oral flecainide and propafenone may offer good suppression of AAs. However, their negative inotropic and pro-arrhythmic characteristics necessitate utmost caution in ACHD patients with HF. These agents are contra-indicated in cases of coronary artery disease, systemic LV dysfunction, and systemic or subpulmonary RV dysfunction.[13] Class III antiarrhythmic agents namely amiodarone, sotalol, and dofetilide offer viable options for managing of arrhythmias in ACHD. Amiodarone is the preferred agent in cases involving heart failure, while sotalol is not advisable when systemic or subpulmonary systolic ventricular dysfunction is present. Dofetilide has been demonstrated to have an effective efficacy in ACHD patients, albeit with a risk of torsade's de pointes in situations marked by prolonged QTc intervals and renal dysfunction. Close monitoring of the QTc interval and careful evaluation of renal function are essential for the safe administration of this agent for arrhythmia suppression.[36,37]

Amiodarone's adverse effects encompass a range of issues, including but not restricted to thyroid dysfunction. Patients with BMI below 21 Kg/m^2, women with cyanotic heart disease, and those who have undergone Fontan palliation are susceptible to amiodarone-induced thyrotoxicosis, which can further worsen HF.[38] Data concerning the use of ibutilide, another class III agent available in intravenous form, suggest it could be a viable option for the acute medical cardioversion of intra-atrial re-entrant tachycardia (IART) or atrial fibrillation in ACHD patients. However, caution is paramount,

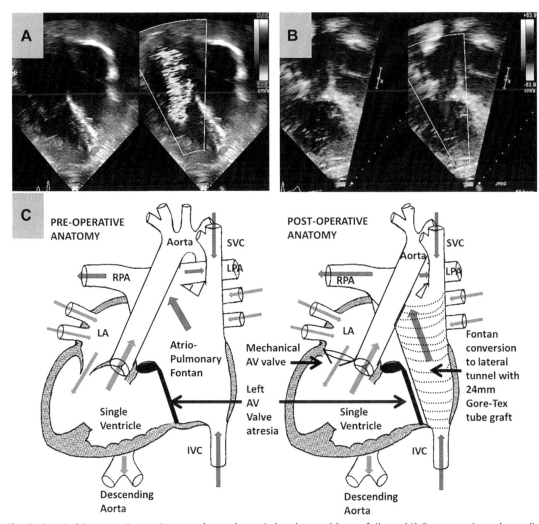

Fig. 3. Surgical intervention to improve hemodynamic burden and heart failure: (A) Pre-operative echocardiogram image demonstrating severely dilated atrium and severe AV valve insufficiency in a patient with atrio-pulmonary Fontan and decompensated heart failure. (B) Post-operative image demonstrating resolution of AV valve insufficiency with mechanical valve replacement. (C) Diagram representing patient's prior to and post-operative anatomy. AV, atrio-ventricular; IVC, inferior vena cava; LA, left atrium; LPA, left pulmonary artery; RPA, right pulmonary artery; SVC, superior vena cava.

necessitating close monitoring of QTc interval and presence of emergency defibrillation resources, due to an associated risk of approximately 4.3% for torsades de pointes. This risk is particularly pronounced in women and African Americans.[13,36,37,39]

Hemodynamic Interventions, arrhythmia surgery: Both mechanical and electrical interactions play a role in the development of arrhythmia in ACHD patients. Interventions aimed at improving hemodynamic load may yield favorable effects on suppressing arrhythmias. In patients with TOF, pulmonary valve replacement (PVR) when indicated has been observed to stabilize QRS duration. When coupled with intraoperative cryoablation to create the lines of blocks across the isthmuses in the RV, the

approach may potentially mitigate the risk of both atrial and ventricular arrhythmias.[40] In a study involving 165 patients with TOF and implantable cardioverter defibrillators (ICD), the incidence of ICD shocks was significantly decreased following PVR.[41] In a study comprising 149 patients, Fontan conversion combined with arrhythmia surgery in meticulously chosen cases of failing atrio-pulmonary Fontan circulation patients exhibited low mortality (2%) and freedom from death and transplant-free survival of 84% at 10 years.[42] In patients undergoing surgery for Fontan revision, Ebstein anomaly, right heart conduit revision, tricuspid valve surgery, left sides valve repair/replacement, and ASD closure, it is reasonable to perform prophylactic arrhythmia surgery (modified right atrial Maze, left atrial Cox Maze III procedure) based on the underlying substrate.[13]

Electrophysiology Interventions: Electrophysiology interventions for arrhythmia management in ACHD encompass both device-based and catheter-based therapies.

Device-based therapy: Arrhythmia management strategies utilizing cardiac implantable electronic devices (CIED) are invaluable tools. The devices are employed for the treatment of bradyarrhythmias, tachycarrhythmias, and the prevention of SCD.

Treatment of Bradyarrhythmia

SND is prevalent in ACHD due to factors such as abnormally formed, absent, or surgically disrupted sinus node. Patients who have undergone the Fontan operation and those who have had atrial switch procedures for D-TGA are especially susceptible to SND (**Table 1**). SND and AAs often coexist and mutually influence each other, initiating and perpetuating a cycle. AAs are present in 40% to 70% of patients upon SND diagnosis.[43] Anti-bradycardia pacing alone has been shown to provide atrial and ventricular arrhythmia suppression in patients with CHD.[44,45] Successful trans-venous pacing can be achieved in patients with atrio-pulmonary or lateral tunnel Fontan procedures (**Fig. 4**).

AV block can manifest spontaneously or as a consequence of surgical intervention. It has the potential to exacerbate HF due to the absence of AV synchrony or a resulting low cardiac output state. Achieving AV synchronous pacing in complex ACHD patients, especially those with Fontan circulation may not be straight forward endeavor. Similarly, patients with intracardiac shunts necessitate careful assessment of defect closure to prevent risk of thromboembolism.

Treatment of Tachyarrhythmia and Prevention of Sudden Cardiac Death

CIED offer anti-tachycardia pacing capabilities that prove beneficial for both atrial and ventricular arrhythmias. SCD is a leading cause of death in ACHD patients. Certain specific ACHD conditions such as TOF and D-transposition of the great arteries (D-TGA) with atrial switch operation have been better studied in terms of predicting or risk stratifying the risk of SCD.[9,46] For patients with TOF at high risk for SCD due to factors like left ventricular dysfunction, extensive ventricular scarring, or an inducible sustained VT-primary prevention, ICDs may be considered.[9] In ACHD patients with systemic left ventricle, an LVEF $\leq$ 35% and New York Heart Association (NYHA) class II or III symptoms meet the criteria for an ICD implantation. It iss important to note that trans-venous ICD implant may not always be feasible. In suitable cases where pacing is unnecessary and QRS duration is not $\geq$ 148 ms, a subcutaneous ICD may be an option.[47,48] The choice between subcutaneous coils and epicardial patches is based on patient's underlying congenital heart defect especially when trans-venous lead placement is not possible (**Fig. 5**).

Cardiac Resynchronization Therapy and Conduction System Pacing

Indications for cardiac resynchronization therapy (CRT) in ACHD can be categorized into dysfunction of the systemic LV, systemic RV, or single ventricle. Class I indications include an LVEF of $\leq$ 35% and a QRS duration of greater than 150 ms with left bundle branch block (LBBB) morphology. For other indications, whether concerning systemic RV, LV,

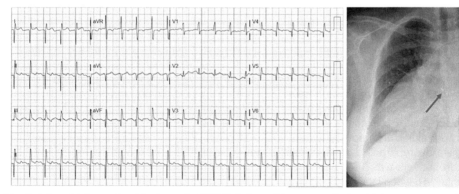

Fig. 4. Intra-atrial re-entrant tachycardia IART (*left image*) in a young lady with heterotaxy syndrome, lateral tunnel Fontan, and sinus node dysfunction managed with anti-arrhythmic drug therapy. A trans-venous atrial lead pacemaker was also implanted (*right image*, indicated by the *red arrow*).

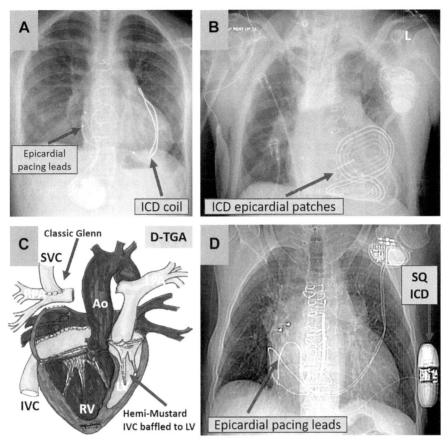

Fig. 5. Epicardial ICD implant in complex ACHD patients. (*A*) Patient with VSD, life-threatening endocarditis, implanted with an epicardial ICD, note the shocking coil looped around the left ventricle. (*B*) Patient with right ventricle to pulmonary artery conduit, severe tricuspid valve insufficiency necessitating replacement, aborted SCD received an epicardial pacemaker along with epicardial shocking patches. (*C*) Anatomic diagram of the patient featured in image D with Hemi-Mutsard repair. (*D*) Patient with D-TGA who underwent Hemi-Mustard operation (classic Glenn anastomosis), this patient received an epicardial CRT-P device and a subcutaneous ICD. Ao, aorta; IVC, inferior vena cava; LV, left ventricle; RPS, right pulmonary artery; RV, right ventricle; SQ ICD, subcutaneous ICD; SVC, superior vena cava.

or single ventricle dysfunction, factors considered include QRS duration greater than 150 ms with right bundle branch block (RBBB), LVEF of ≤ 35% or > 35% with NYHA II–IV symptoms, or pacing needs of greater than 40%.[13] In pediatric and CHD patients experiencing symptomatic systolic HF with electrical dyssynchrony, CRT has been demonstrated to enhance heart transplant–free survival.[49]

Given the anatomic complexities inherent in CHD, the strategy for placing CRT leads must often be tailored to the specific anatomy. In patients with CCTGA combined with heart block, primary biventricular pacing has demonstrated efficacy in preventing systemic ventricular dysfunction or even enhancing systemic ventricular function, particularly in cases previously managed with univentricular

pacing.[50] In appropriately chosen patients presenting with systemic RV dysfunction and pacing-induced dyssynchrony, CRT consistently led to improvement in QRS duration and NYHA functional status. Although there was only a marginal increase in systemic RV function.[51] Another study demonstrated that CRT resulted in improved late hemodynamic and functional status in CHD patients with systemic LV and those with systemic unbalanced or single ventricles experiencing dyssynchrony in the systemic ventricle. However, while an acute CRT effect was not observed, it could not ensure long-term benefits for patients with systemic RV.[52]

Physiologic or conduction system pacing (CSP), which encompasses His bundle pacing and left bundle pacing (LBP), is increasingly acknowledged for its role in preventing and alleviating

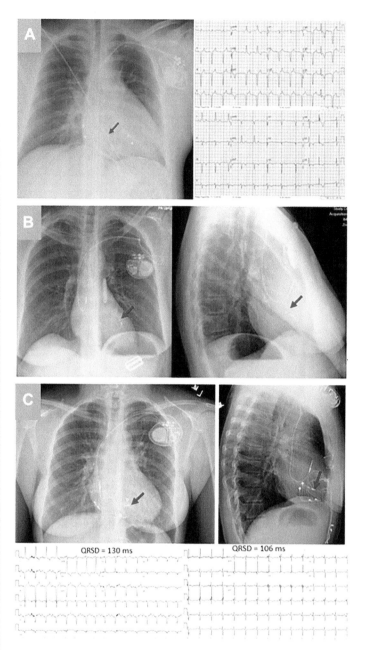

Fig. 6. Conduction system pacing in ACHD. (*A*) Depicting a case of repaired AV canal defect with pacing- induced cardiomyopathy. His bundle pacing (*red arrow*) was utilized achieving a narrow QRS and improved ventricular function. (*B*) Left bundle pacing (*red arrow*) in a patient with heart block after cone operation for Ebstein anomaly of the tricuspid valve. (*C*) Left bundle pacing (*red arrow*) in a patient with history of ventricular septal defect, heart block who underwent upgrade of an epicardial dual chamber to a trans-venous system (QRS duration 130 ms → 106 ms).

HF.[53] Abnormal or displaced conduction system, AV node/His bundle location in CHD may pose challenges with conduction system localization and CSP in ACHD patients. In CHD, abnormal or displaced conduction systems, as well as variations in AV node/His bundle location, can present challenges in localizing the conduction system and implementing CSP in ACHD patients. It is important to note that CSP may not be suitable for all forms of ACHD, including those who have undergone Fontan palliation. With careful patient selection and understanding of the conduction system's location in ACHD patients, permanent CSP can both be safe and feasible[54] (**Fig. 6**).

CATHETER-BASED ELECTROPHYSIOLOGY THERAPIES IN ADULT CONGENITAL HEART DISEASE
Catheter Ablation of Atrial Arrhythmia

AAs in ACHD patients frequently prove resistant to medical treatment and prolonged medication

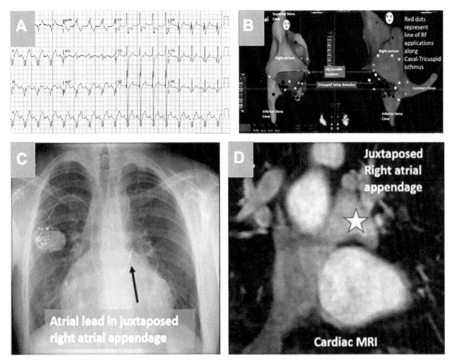

Fig. 7. Patient is an 18-year-old male with D-TGA, mesocardia, juxtaposed right atrial appendage. (*A*) Depicts intra-atrial reentrant tachycardia with 2:1 AV conduction. (*B*) Features the electro-anatomic map displaying ablation lesions. (*C*) Displays the pacing lead correctly positioned in the juxtaposed right atrial appendage. (*D*) Representation of the anatomy as demonstrated by cardiac MRI. The *yellow star* in the image represents the juxtaposed right atrial appendage.

usage may lead to unfavorable side effects. Catheter Ablation of AA offers an excellent success at experienced hands and early ablation strategies can be considered[13,55]. Complexity of CHD plays a significant role in determining the success and recurrence rates of ablation procedures. In the context of ACHD patients, the use of irrigated tip radiofrequency ablation catheters tends to yield improved success rates [13] In specific forms of CHD, such as atrial switch operation for D-TGA or Fontan palliated patients, special techniques like retrograde approaches or baffle punctures may be necessary.[56,57] Caval-tricuspid atrial–dependent flutter and atriotomy sites are frequent sites of IART occurrences in ACHD conditions like TOF and D-TGA following atrial switch operations.[9] Familiarity with surgical repair and the anticipated scar site can significantly aid electrophysiologists for ablation therapies. While catheter ablation for atrial fibrillation is viable in patients with CHD, it is important to note that the likelihood of achieving lasting success is diminished in patients with anatomically intricate conditions.[58] In certain scenarios, a combined approach involving atrial flutter ablation and

pacemaker implantation may become necessary when tachycardia-bradycardia syndrome coexists (**Fig. 7**).

Catheter Ablation of Ventricular Arrhythmia

Ventricular arrhythmia substrates have been notably elucidated in specific forms of ACHD, such as TOF and Ebstein anomaly of the tricuspid valve.[9,59,60] Reported success rates for catheter ablation of ventricular arrhythmias have ranged from 57% to 70%. However, recurrence rates can be as high as 40%.[61,62] Pre-operative electrophysiology studies prior to Cone operation are recommended and the importance of these studies is increasingly recognized in patients with TOF before undergoing pulmonary valve replacement.[63] Frequent ventricular ectopy can also cause ventricular dysfunction. In cases where it is identified as a culprit, ectopy ablation can be perused. For patients with pre-existing ICDs receiving frequent appropriate shocks, catheter ablation should be undertaken to reduce ICD shocks along with optimization of pharmacologic therapy.

SUMMARY

In ACHD patients, the coexistence of arrhythmias and HF often displays an intricate interplay. This interrelationship is associated with heightened morbidity and mortality. The specific underlying CHD condition guides the choice of management strategies. Effective management strategies encompass a range of interventions, including pharmacotherapy for both arrhythmias and HF, transcatheter or surgical hemodynamic optimization, the utilization of CIEDs, and catheter ablation of arrhythmias.

CLINICS CARE POINTS

- Proactively identify and address arrhythmias in adults with congenital heart disease (ACHD).
- Explore arrhythmias as a potential cause of heart failure in ACHD patients, and reciprocally, consider heart failure exacerbation as a trigger for arrhythmia development.
- Recognize that the management of arrhythmias or heart failure in the ACHD population may necessitate tailored approaches, as conventional heart failure strategies may not consistently yield optimal results. Individualized care is paramount in this context.

DISCLOSURE

Both authors have nothing to disclose.

REFERENCES

1. Diller GP, Kempny A, Alonso-Gonzalez R, et al. Survival prospects and circumstances of death in contemporary adult congenital heart disease patients under follow-up at a large tertiary centre. Circulation 2015;132(22):2118–25.
2. Engelings CC, Helm PC, Abdul-Khaliq H, et al. Cause of death in adults with congenital heart disease - an analysis of the German National Register for congenital heart defects. Int J Cardiol 2016; 211:31–6.
3. Norozi K, Wessel A, Alpers V, et al. Incidence and risk distribution of heart failure in adolescents and adults with congenital heart disease after cardiac surgery. Am J Cardiol 2006;97(8):1238–43.
4. Yu C, Moore BM, Kotchetkova I, et al. Causes of death in a contemporary adult congenital heart disease cohort. Heart 2018;104(20):1678–82.
5. Zomer AC, Vaartjes I, Uiterwaal CS, et al. Circumstances of death in adult congenital heart disease. Int J Cardiol 2012;154(2):168–72.
6. Bouchardy J, Therrien J, Pilote L, et al. Atrial arrhythmias in adults with congenital heart disease. Circulation 2009;120(17):1679–86.
7. Lindsay I, Moore JP. Cardiac Arrhythmias in Adults With Congenital Heart Disease: Scope, Specific Problems, and Management. Curr Treat Options Cardiovasc Med 2015;17(12):56.
8. Egbe AC, Najam M, Banala K, et al. Impact of atrial arrhythmia on survival in adults with tetralogy of fallot. Am Heart J 2019;218:1–7.
9. Krieger EV, Zeppenfeld K, DeWitt ES, et al. Arrhythmias in repaired tetralogy of fallot: a scientific statement from the American Heart Association. Circ Arrhythm Electrophysiol 2022;15(11):e000084.
10. Giannakoulas G, Dimopoulos K, Yuksel S, et al. Atrial tachyarrhythmias late after Fontan operation are related to increase in mortality and hospitalization. Int J Cardiol 2012;157(2):221–6.
11. Khairy P, Van Hare GF, Balaji S, et al. PACES/HRS expert consensus statement on the recognition and management of arrhythmias in adult congenital heart disease: developed in partnership between the Pediatric and Congenital Electrophysiology Society (PACES) and the Heart Rhythm Society (HRS). Endorsed by the governing bodies of PACES, HRS, the American College of Cardiology (ACC), the American Heart Association (AHA), the European Heart Rhythm Association (EHRA), the Canadian Heart Rhythm Society (CHRS), and the International Society for Adult Congenital Heart Disease (ISACHD). Can J Cardiol 2014;30(10):e1–63.
12. Moore JP, Marelli A, Burchill LJ, et al. Management of heart failure with arrhythmia in adults with congenital heart disease: JACC state-of-the-art review. J Am Coll Cardiol 2022;80(23):2224–38.
13. Khairy P, Van Hare GF, Balaji S, et al. PACES/HRS expert consensus statement on the recognition and management of arrhythmias in adult congenital heart disease: developed in partnership between the Pediatric and Congenital Electrophysiology Society (PACES) and the Heart Rhythm Society (HRS). Endorsed by the governing bodies of PACES, HRS, the American College of Cardiology (ACC), the American Heart Association (AHA), the European Heart Rhythm Association (EHRA), the Canadian Heart Rhythm Society (CHRS), and the International Society for Adult. Heart rhythm 2014;11(10). e102–65.
14. Escudero C, Khairy P, Sanatani S. Electrophysiologic considerations in congenital heart disease and their relationship to heart failure. Can J Cardiol 2013; 29(7). https://doi.org/10.1016/j.cjca.2013.02.016.
15. Bessière F, Mondésert B, Chaix MA, et al. Arrhythmias in adults with congenital heart disease and heart failure. Heart Rhythm O2 2021;2(6):744–53.

16. Anabtawi A, Mondragon J, Dodendorf D, et al. Late-stage left ventricular dysfunction in adult survivors of tetralogy of Fallot repair in childhood. Open Heart 2017;4(2). https://doi.org/10.1136/openhrt-2017-000690.

17. Egbe AC, Adigun R, Anand V, et al. Left ventricular systolic dysfunction and cardiovascular outcomes in tetralogy of fallot: systematic review and meta-analysis. Can J Cardiol 2019;35(12):1784–90.

18. Aboulhosn JA, Lluri G, Gurvitz MZ, et al. Left and right ventricular diastolic function in adults with surgically repaired tetralogy of Fallot: a multi-institutional study. Can J Cardiol 2013;29(7):866–72.

19. Graham TP Jr, Bernard YD, Mellen BG, et al. Long-term outcome in congenitally corrected transposition of the great arteries: a multi-institutional study. J Am Coll Cardiol 2000;36(1):255–61.

20. Moore BM, Medi C, McGuire MA, et al. Pacing-associated cardiomyopathy in adult congenital heart disease. Open Heart 2020;7(2). https://doi.org/10.1136/openhrt-2020-001374.

21. Andrade L, Carazo M, Wu F, et al. Mechanisms for heart failure in systemic right ventricle. Heart Fail Rev 2020;25(4). https://doi.org/10.1007/s10741-019-09902-1.

22. Khairy P, Van Hare GF. Catheter ablation in transposition of the great arteries with Mustard or Senning baffles. Heart Rhythm 2009;6(2). https://doi.org/10.1016/j.hrthm.2008.11.022.

23. Khairy P, Harris L, Landzberg MJ, et al. Sudden death and defibrillators in transposition of the great arteries with intra-atrial baffles: a multicenter study. Circ Arrhythm Electrophysiol 2008;1(4):250–7.

24. Kammeraad JA, Van Deurzen CH, Sreeram N, et al. Predictors of sudden cardiac death after Mustard or Senning repair for transposition of the great arteries. Journal of the American College of Cardiology 2004; 44(5). 1095–102.

25. Haddad F, Hunt SA, Rosenthal DN, et al. Right ventricular function in cardiovascular disease, part I: Anatomy, physiology, aging, and functional assessment of the right ventricle. Circulation 2008;117(11). https://doi.org/10.1161/CIRCULATIONAHA.107.653576.

26. Kaye GC, Astridge P, Perrins J. Tachycardia recognition and diagnosis from changes in right atrial pressure waveform–a feasibility study. Pacing Clin Electrophysiol 1991;14(9):1384–92.

27. Perrin N, Dore A, van de Bruaene A, et al. The fontan circulation: from ideal to failing hemodynamics and drug therapies for optimization. Can J Cardiol 2022;38(7):1059–71.

28. Rychik J, Veldtman G, Rand E, et al. The precarious state of the liver after a fontan operation: summary of a multidisciplinary symposium. Pediatr Cardiol 2012; 33(7):1001–12.

29. Khairy P, Poirier N, Mercier LA. Univentricular heart. Circulation 2007;115(6). https://doi.org/10.1161/CIRCULATIONAHA.105.592378.

30. Piran S, Veldtman G, Siu S, et al. Heart failure and ventricular dysfunction in patients with single or systemic right ventricles. Circulation 2002;105(10). https://doi.org/10.1161/hc1002.105182.

31. Deal BJ. Late Arrhythmias Following Fontan Surgery. World J Pediatr Congenit Heart Surg 2012;3(2): 194–200.

32. Giacone HM, Chubb H, Dubin AM, et al. Outcomes after development of ventricular arrhythmias in single ventricular heart disease patients with fontan palliation. Circ Arrhythm Electrophysiol 2023;16(6): e011143.

33. Torp-Pedersen C, Poole-Wilson PA, Swedberg K, et al. Effects of metoprolol and carvedilol on cause-specific mortality and morbidity in patients with chronic heart failure–COMET. Am Heart J 2005;149(2):370–6.

34. Hjalmarson Å, Fagerberg B. MERIT-HF mortality and morbidity data. Basic Research in Cardiology 2000; 95(1). https://doi.org/10.1007/s003950070017.

35. Guerra F, Pimpini L, Flori M, et al. Sacubitril/valsartan reduces atrial fibrillation and supraventricular arrhythmias in patients with HFrEF and remote monitoring: preliminary data from the SAVE THE RHYTHM. Eur Heart J 2020;41:ehaa946–0926.

36. Wells R, Khairy P, Harris L, et al. Dofetilide for atrial arrhythmias in congenital heart disease: A multicenter study. PACE - Pacing and Clinical Electrophysiology 2009;32(10). https://doi.org/10.1111/j.1540-8159.2009.02479.x.

37. El-Assaad I, Al-Kindi SG, Abraham J, et al. Use of dofetilide in adult patients with atrial arrhythmias and congenital heart disease: a PACES collaborative study. Heart Rhythm 2016;13(10):2034–9.

38. Kawada S, Chakraborty P, Roche L, et al. Role of amiodarone in the management of atrial arrhythmias in adult Fontan patients. Heart 2021;107(13):1062–8.

39. Dasgupta S, Dave I, Whitehill R, et al. Chemical cardioversion of atrial flutter and fibrillation in the pediatric population with Ibutilide. PACE - Pacing and Clinical Electrophysiology 2020;43(3). https://doi.org/10.1111/pace.13890.

40. Therrien J, Siu SC, Harris L, et al. Impact of pulmonary valve replacement on arrhythmia propensity late after repair of tetralogy of Fallot. Circulation 2001;103(20):2489–94.

41. Bessière F, Gardey K, Bouzeman A, et al. Impact of pulmonary valve replacement on ventricular arrhythmias in patients with tetralogy of fallot and implantable cardioverter-defibrillator. JACC Clin Electrophysiol 2021;7(10):1285–93.

42. Backer CL, Mavroudis C. 149 Fontan Conversions. Methodist Debakey Cardiovasc J 2019;15(2). https://doi.org/10.14797/mdcj-15-2-105.

43. John RM, Kumar S. Sinus Node and Atrial Arrhythmias. Circulation 2016;133(19):1892–900. https://doi.org/10.1161/CIRCULATIONAHA.116.018011.

44. Kramer CC, Maldonado JR, Olson MD, et al. Safety and efficacy of atrial antitachycardia pacing in congenital heart disease. Heart Rhythm 2018;15(4). https://doi.org/10.1016/j.hrthm.2017.12.016.

45. Kamp AN, Lapage MJ, Serwer GA, et al. Antitachycardia pacemakers in congenital heart disease. Congenit Heart Dis 2015;10(2). https://doi.org/10.1111/chd.12230.

46. Broberg CS, van Dissel A, Minnier J, et al. Long-term outcomes after atrial switch operation for transposition of the great arteries. J Am Coll Cardiol 2022;80(10):951–63.

47. Sarubbi B, Correra A, Colonna D, et al. Subcutaneous implantable cardioverter defibrillator in complex adult congenital heart disease. Results from the S-ICD "Monaldi Care" registry. IJC Congenital Heart Disease 2021;3:100091.

48. Zormpas C, Silber-Peest AS, Eiringhaus J, et al. Eligibility for subcutaneous implantable cardioverter-defibrillator in adults with congenital heart disease. ESC Heart Fail 2021;8(2):1502–8.

49. Chubb H, Rosenthal DN, Almond CS, et al. Impact of cardiac resynchronization therapy on heart transplant-free survival in pediatric and congenital heart disease patients. Circ Arrhythm Electrophysiol 2020;13(4):e007925.

50. Hofferberth SC, Alexander ME, Mah DY, et al. Impact of pacing on systemic ventricular function in L-transposition of the great arteries. J Thorac Cardiovasc Surg 2016;151(1):131–8.

51. Kharbanda RK, Moore JP, Taverne YJHJ, et al. Cardiac resynchronization therapy for the failing systemic right ventricle: A systematic review. Int J Cardiol 2020;318:74–81.

52. Sakaguchi H, Miyazaki A, Yamada O, et al. Cardiac resynchronization therapy for various systemic ventricular morphologies in patients with congenital heart disease. Circ J 2015;79(3):649–55.

53. Chung M.K., Patton K.K., Lau C.P., et al., 2023 HRS/APHRS/LAHRS guideline on cardiac physiologic pacing for the avoidance and mitigation of heart failure. Heart Rhythm. 2023;20(9):e17-e91.

54. Cano Ó, Dandamudi G, Schaller RD, et al. Safety and feasibility of conduction system pacing in patients with congenital heart disease. J Cardiovasc Electrophysiol 2021;32(10):2692–703.

55. Roca-Luque I, Rivas-Gándara N, Dos Subirà L, et al. Long-term follow-up after ablation of intra-atrial re-entrant tachycardia in patients with congenital heart disease: types and predictors of recurrence. JACC Clin Electrophysiol 2018;4(6):771–80.

56. Correa R, Walsh EP, Alexander ME, et al. Transbaffle mapping and ablation for atrial tachycardias after mustard, senning, or Fontan operations. J Am Heart Assoc 2013;2(5):e000325.

57. Jones DG, Jarman JWE, Lyne JC, et al. The safety and efficacy of trans-baffle puncture to enable catheter ablation of a trial tachycardias following the Mustard procedure: A single centre experience and literature review. Int J Cardiol 2013;168(2). https://doi.org/10.1016/j.ijcard.2012.11.047.

58. Liang JJ, Frankel DS, Parikh V, et al. Safety and outcomes of catheter ablation for atrial fibrillation in adults with congenital heart disease: a multicenter registry study. Heart Rhythm 2019;16(6):846–52.

59. Moore JP, Shannon KM, Gallotti RG, et al. Catheter ablation of ventricular arrhythmia for ebstein's anomaly in unoperated and post-surgical patients. JACC Clin Electrophysiol 2018;4(10):1300–7.

60. Zeppenfeld K, Schalij MJ, Bartelings MM, et al. Catheter ablation of ventricular tachycardia after repair of congenital heart disease: electroanatomic identification of the critical right ventricular isthmus. Circulation 2007;116(20):2241–52.

61. Furushima H, Chinushi M, Sugiura H, et al. Ventricular tachycardia late after repair of congenital heart disease: efficacy of combination therapy with radiofrequency catheter ablation and class III antiarrhythmic agents and long-term outcome. J Electrocardiol 2006;39(2):219–24.

62. Morwood JG, Triedman JK, Berul CI, et al. Radiofrequency catheter ablation of ventricular tachycardia in children and young adults with congenital heart disease. Heart Rhythm 2004;1(3):301–8.

63. Bouyer B, Jalal Z, Daniel Ramirez F, et al. Electrophysiological study prior to planned pulmonary valve replacement in patients with repaired tetralogy of Fallot. J Cardiovasc Electrophysiol 2023;34(6):1395–404.

The Role of Multimodality Imaging in the Evaluation of Heart Failure and Surgical Transplant Planning of Patients with Adult Congenital Heart Disease

Valeria E. Duarte, MD, MPH[a],*, Saurabh Rajpal, MD[b]

KEYWORDS

- Adult congenital heart disease • Heart failure • Transplant • Congenital imaging • Cardiac MRI
- Cardiac CT • Echocardiography

KEY POINTS

- Patients with adult congenital heart disease (ACHD) need routine surveillance imaging to identify long-term complications and residual lesions that might be targets for optimization.
- Longitudinal imaging in patients with ACHD is key for the timely identification of patients requiring evaluation for advanced therapies.
- Multimodality imaging plays an important role in preoperative planning for surgery, including transplantation and mechanical support.
- Imaging in ACHD patients should performed at centers with expertise, and the imaging protocols should be tailored to the specific condition and each patient's unique native and postsurgical anatomy.

INTRODUCTION

Cardiac imaging is pivotal in evaluating ventricular function and residual lesions that might be targets for clinical optimization in patients with adult congenital heart disease (ACHD). In addition, longitudinal cardiac imaging is critical in the assessment of the effects of treatment and timely identification of patients who would benefit from consideration for advanced heart failure therapies. The guidelines recommend routine imaging surveillance, with the frequency and modality of imaging varying according to specific conditions.[1] For instance, in individuals with simple defects, a transthoracic echocardiogram (TTE) every 3 years suffices, whereas for asymptomatic adults with repaired tetralogy of Fallot, D-loop transposition of the great arteries (TGA) following arterial switch operation, Rastelli procedure, or atrial switch operation, as well as those with congenitally corrected TGA (ccTGA) or single ventricle after Fontan procedure without or with mild sequelae, a yearly TTE in conjunction with cardiac magnetic resonance (CMR) and cardiac computed tomography (CCT) every 2 to 5 years is recommended for routine surveillance. In adults with congenital heart disease (CHD) who present with clinical heart

a Department of Cardiology, Houston Methodist DeBakey Heart and Vascular Center, 6550 Fannin St, Smith Tower suite 1801, Houston, TX 77030, USA; b Department of Cardiology, Division of Cardiovascular Medicine, The Ohio State University, 473 W 12th Avenue, Davis Heart and Lung Research Institute, Columbus, OH 43210, USA
* Corresponding author.
E-mail address: vduarte@houstonmethodist.org

Heart Failure Clin 20 (2024) 189–198
https://doi.org/10.1016/j.hfc.2024.01.002
1551-7136/24/© 2024 Elsevier Inc. All rights reserved.

failure, periodic imaging through TTE, CMR, and CCT is considered appropriate for the evaluation of valvular and ventricular function.[1,2] In all patients undergoing evaluation with cardiac imaging, it is critical to know the patient's native anatomy and surgical history in detail in order to protocol the study appropriately and answer all the clinical questions. The authors will briefly highlight the utility and diagnostic yield of different modalities, review pertinent considerations for special populations, and focus on imaging for transplant planning, as the literature on this topic is limited.

Echocardiography

Echocardiography is the initial modality for evaluating CHD anatomy, hemodynamics, ventricular, and valvular function. It is cost-effective, reproducible, and more accessible than other modalities. It is essential to measure the gradients across obstructive lesions (valve stenosis, left ventricular outflow tract [LVOT] and right ventricular outflow tract [RVOT] obstruction, supramitral ring, coarctation, supravalvar pulmonary stenosis [supra-PS] and supravalvular aortic stenosis [supra-AS], and branch pulmonary artery [PA] stenosis), as well to assess regurgitant valve lesions, and for hemodynamic assessment and estimation of the estimate right ventricle (RV) systolic pressure. Patency of other vascular structures such as superior vena cava (SVC), inferior vena cava (IVC) (native or baffles), pulmonary veins (native and baffles), Fontan conduit, and fenestration is also reliable by echocardiography. Still, it requires a highly trained congenital sonographer and cardiac imager. Transesophageal echocardiography (TEE) is a useful technique in certain situations where transthoracic images are challenging to interpret due to poor acoustic windows and in certain conditions such as sinus venosus defects or anomalous pulmonary venous return, where important information can be missed by TTE alone.

Ventricular function assessment
Systolic and diastolic ventricular dysfunction should be comprehensive and frequently require nonconventional views. Volumetric assessment with 3-dimensional (3D) technology is essential. Cardiac strain is gaining relevance in ACHD patients and can be helpful when monitoring a patient longitudinally. RV size and function assessment can be limited in some cases, particularly in patients with systemic RVs (congenitally corrected transposition, d-loop transposition status after atrial switch) and univentricular hearts. In palliate univentricular hearts, it is essential to identify the ventricular morphology of the single

ventricle, as it has prognostic implications. Elements that help identify a morphologic RV are chordal attachments to the septum, a moderator band, no fibrous continuity between the aortic and atrioventricular (AV) valves, and increased trabeculations.[3] Diastolic assessment with spectral and tissue Doppler is recommended. Notably, in patients with palliated univentricular hearts, spectral Doppler measurements can be abnormal due to low preload.[3] Doppler-based tissue velocity measurements (tissue Doppler) should be part of the hemodynamic assessment of ventricular filling pressures. Speckle tracking echocardiography has been expanding its clinical applications and can be helpful to for longitudinal follow-up of ACHD patients.[4–6]

Obstructive lesions
Measuring the gradients across obstructive lesions is very important. Valvular stenosis should be assessed as specified by current guidelines. Other obstructive lesions that should be carefully evaluated include LVOT, and RVOT obstruction, supramitral ring, coarctation of the aorta, supra-PS and supra-AS, branch PA stenosis, as well as to assess regurgitant valve lesions and perform a hemodynamic assessment and estimation of the estimated RV systolic pressure.

Vascular structures
The patency of major vascular structures such as SVC, IVC (native or baffles), pulmonary veins (native and baffles), Fontan conduit, and fenestration is also reliable by echocardiography but require a highly trained congenital imaging team (sonographer/cardiologist).

Dextrocardia, mesocardia, situs inversus, and heterotaxy syndromes can present significant challenges during imaging acquisition. Dedicated and comprehensive training of the echocardiographer is critical to obtaining a diagnostic study despite these challenges.

Transesophageal echocardiography
TEE can be useful where transthoracic echocardiographic windows are challenging. Specifically TEE is useful in assessments of small shunts, sinus venosus or coronary sinus defects, anomalous pulmonary venous return or connection, evaluation of systemic AV valve in with systemic RV (congenitally corrected transposition, d-loop transposition status after atrial switch and Fontan circulation), assessment of eccentric jets, evaluation of Fontan fenestration, and assessment of ventricular function where cross-sectional imaging is not feasible (significant metallic artifact, non-MRI compatible pacemakers and defibrillators, abandoned epicardial leads) or available. In

addition, TEE is the modality of choice to guide transcatheter valve interventions.

Cross-Sectional Imaging

Both CMR and CCT provide a 3D assessment of anatomy, volume, and function, as well as a comprehensive assessment of vascular structures in patients with ACHD. Each modality has its benefits and challenges.

Cardiac MRI

CMR is a comprehensive imaging modality that is helpful in the cross-sectional assessment of anatomy, function, hemodynamics, and tissue characterization and is the gold standard modality for the volumetric and functional evaluation of the ventricles. CMR is not as available as echocardiography and computed tomography, and it requires a high level of expertise and understanding of CHD for protocoling, image acquisition, and interpretation; therefore, congenital CMR should preferably be performed at specialized ACHD centers. It does not involve radiation exposure. Metallic artifacts due to stents, coils, valve prostheses, sternotomy wires, pacemakers, and defibrillators might decrease imaging quality and the ability to perform flow assessment. CMR studies have a long acquisition time and can be particularly lengthy in patients with CHD. Symptomatic patients might have difficulties tolerating the supine position for a prolonged period. Gadolinium-based agents are the most frequently used contrast agents for CMR angiography and late gadolinium enhancement (LGE) assessment. LGE is particularly useful in the evaluation of myocardial scar in patients with heart failure and arrhythmias. Patients with a single ventricle can also have LGE due to endocardial fibroelastosis . Ferumoxytol-enhanced CMR is increasingly reported as a good alternative, particularly in patients with renal dysfunction. Another added benefit of ferumoxytol as a contrast agent is its prolonged intravascular residence time of more than 12 hours due to its size and carbohydrate coating.[7,8] This feature might help optimize vascular assessment, including collateral vessels. 3D whole heart steady-state free precession provides a reliable 3D dataset to characterize intracardiac and extracardiac structures without requiring contrast administration. It prolongs scan time, so all patients might not tolerate it. Another strength of CMR is the identification of thrombus in the Fontan circulation.

Phase-contrast assessment (2-dimensional flow CMR) is the most used technology to evaluate direction, velocity, and quantify flow across valves, vessels, and cardiac structures, measure regurgitant volumes, and assess the ratio of pulmonary blood flow (Qp) to systemic blood flow (Qs) (Qp: Qs), amongst many other applications. CMR contributes to the assessment of collateral burden. Assessment of SVC and IVC, branch PA, pulmonary veins, and aortic forward flow can help identify the collateral burden and predict the location of the collaterals by flow difference calculations. This is helpful to plan for cardiac catheterization and potential coiling of collaterals to decrease surgical bleeding risk. To optimize accuracy, the velocity encoding (VENC) needs to be adjusted (lowered) for the systemic and pulmonary veins and branch pulmonary arteries in patients with Fontan circulation.

Four-dimensional (4D) flow CMR is time-resolved phase-contrast CMR with flow-encoding in all 3 spatial directions. With this technology, 3D volumetric images are combined with 3D VENC throughout the cardiac cycle. Using 4D-flow CMR, qualification and quantification of flow over an entire volume can be obtained, in contrast to conventional 2-dimensional (2D)-PC CMR by which only basic flow parameters can be measured in a single 2D plane in one direction. Therefore, it allows a comprehensive and accurate flow assessment in a single free-breathing acquisition. It provides the ability to obtain data retrospectively, making protocoling less cumbersome.[9,10]

Cardiac computed tomography

CCT provides excellent spatial resolution imaging with a single breath hold during the first pass of contrast bolus. Imaging acquisition is fast and easily tolerated by patients. Newer generation dual-source scanners have helped decrease scan time and radiation dose. Metallic artifacts are much less prominent than with CMR and minimal in some cases. CCT provides anatomic assessment and is critical for surgical planning. Ventricular volumes and function can be accurately assessed, as well as valvular area and regurgitant orifice. It is particularly relevant in patients who are unable to undergo cardiac CMR due to noncompatible devices, abandoned leads, and claustrophobia. Noncontrast CCT is very helpful in identifying calcification of vascular structures and pericardial calcification.

CCT is the preferred modality for coronary imaging. This is particularly important in patients who underwent coronary manipulation like in the arterial switch, Bentall, and Ross procedure, in whom myocardial ischemia may be an underlying cause of ventricular dysfunction. Coronary evaluation is also essential for patients with coronary anomalies, frequently seen in tetralogy of Fallot and D-loop TGA, conditions such as pulmonary atresia-intact ventricular septum where it is essential to identify RV-dependent circulation.

With the advancement of transcatheter options for CHD, CCT is critical in the planning of transcatheter pulmonary valve replacement in patients with pulmonary valve disease associated with RV enlargement and/or dysfunction. In addition, mitral and tricuspid (subpulmonic or systemic) interventions might be considered to optimize ACHD patients, and CT is critical for procedural planning.[11–13]

CCT for surgical transplant planning needs to be protocoled appropriately to answer all the clinical questions. Extended coverage is recommended, including the innominate vein and branches of the aorta, to the diaphragm and hepatic veins.

CCT in patients with Fontan circulation poses challenges, as detailed in the Fontan imaging section.

3D printing can bring additional value in cases with challenging anatomies, with unusual spatial arrangement of the heart and vascular structures that might lead to challenges at the time of the anastomosis. These can be obtained using both a CT angiography and a CMR dataset.[14]

Special Populations

Preoperative and pretransplant imaging assessment in adult congenital heart disease patients

ACHD patients present transplant surgeons with a myriad of challenges related to native and postsurgical anatomic complexity. Moreover, most ACHD patients have had several operations by the time they are referred for transplant. They may present challenges in several options of the transplant surgery, including reentry, adhesions, collateral vessels that increase bleeding risk, need for vascular reconstruction, need for repair of uncorrected defects, challenges at the time of anastomosis with the donor organs, amongst others. The added complexity is associated with longer surgeries and longer ischemic times for the donor organs. This should be carefully considered, as it might affect strategies at the time of donor selection (ie, travel distance) given the anticipated prolonged ischemic time.

Re-entry strategy planning The recognition of adhesions of cardiovascular structures to the sternum is critical to planning the cannulation strategy. Not infrequently, the RV, the aorta, or RV to PA (RV-PA) conduits (in patients with Rastelli, truncus repair, and pulmonary atresia) adhere to the sternum (**Fig. 1**). In these cases, peripheral cannulation might be preferred. It is important to assess the femoral, axillary, and subclavian vessel patency for planning. Postsurgical adhesions that

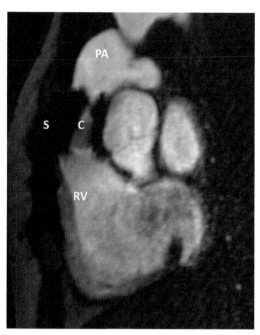

Fig. 1. Cardiac magnetic resonance showing right ventricle-to-pulmonary artery (RV-PA) conduit adhered to the sternum in a patient with prior Ross procedure for congenital aortic stenosis and Melody valve implantation. C, RV-PA conduit; PA, pulmonary artery; RV, right ventricle; S, sternum.

might interfere with cannulation, such as SVC-aortic adhesions, are also of importance.

Vascular assessment From a pretransplant planning perspective, performing a comprehensive evaluation of the vascular anatomy is important. This can be done with CMR and CCT.

- Systemic veins. SVC size, patency, and need for reconstruction, particularly in patients with Glenn, Fontan, and atrial switch, need to be specified. In patients with persistent left SVC, reporting the presence or absence of a bridging vein and its size is pertinent, as this has operative implications. In the presence of a sizable bridging vein, the left SVC can potentially be ligated distal to the bridging vein at the time of transplant. In the absence of a bridging vein, a biatrial transplant, anastomosis of the left SVC to the donor heart's atrial appendage, or the donor's innominate vein are possibilities. The latter requires harvesting of the donor's left innominate vein at the time of organ procurement. IVC assessment is essential; measurement of the distance between the anastomosis with the Fontan conduit or baffle, as well as the presence and severity of calcification that could make the vessel more friable and thus anastomosis more complex, should be assessed. In patients with heterotaxy, discontinuous IVC with azygos continuation who have undergone a Kawashima, and those with a hepatic vein to azygos conduit may need extensive vascular reconstruction, with added surgical complexity and prolonging the duration of the operation.

- Pulmonary veins. Abnormal pulmonary vein anatomy, as in patients with hypoplastic lungs or repaired total anomalous pulmonary vein return, needs careful consideration to plan vascular anastomosis.
- Aorta and branches. Aortic root, ascending aorta, and arch reconstruction might be necessary during transplant. Examples are aneurysmal dilation, arch hypoplasia, patients with repaired truncus, or patients with a Damus Kaye Stansel procedure (**Fig. 2**A). Accurate measurement of the different segments of the aorta is important to determine the need and size of interposition grafts and to optimize the extent of procurement. Aortic branching pattern and variants such as bovine trunk and aberrant subclavian origin should be characterized. Patency of the subclavian artery in patients with previous Blalock-Taussig shunt or coarctation repair should be noted (**Fig. 2**B).

- Patent ductus arteriosus (PDA) adds additional complexity at the time of heart or heart and lung transplantation, as it requires closure of the PDA ostium in the aorta with circulatory arrest at the time of transplantation. Nonconventional cannulation strategies may be considered to preserve cerebral perfusion during circulatory arrest (ie, cannulation of the right axillary artery with temporal occlusion of the right innominate artery). Unrepaired PDAs in adults can have significant calcification that needs to be reported as it makes surgical ligation challenging and might need a vascular flap or patch repair.
- Pulmonary arteries. Patients with Fontan circulations and RV-PA conduits, hypoplastic or stented branch pulmonary arteries will require vascular reconstruction (**Fig. 2**C). Pulmonary arterio-venous malformations should be noted as well.
- Collateral vessels. Bleeding complications are frequent in ACHD transplants, and numerous collateral vessels that develop in certain

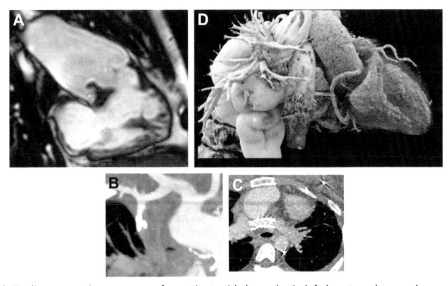

Fig. 2. (A) Cardiac magnetic resonance of a patient with hypoplastic left heart syndrome who underwent a Damus Kaye Stansel (DKS) procedure and Fontan palliation. (*asterisk*) points to the hypoplastic native aortic root and (*dagger*) points to the neo-aortic root that have been anastomosed. The ascending aorta is severely dilated. This patient will need aortic reconstruction at the time of transplant. (B) Cardiac computed tomography in a patient with single ventricle physiology status after Fontan palliation for heart and liver transplantation planning. A bovine trunk branching pattern of the aortic arch is noted. (*asterisk*) points an occluded right-sided Blalock-Taussig shunt. Ao, aortic arch; LC, left carotid artery; RC, right carotid artery; RSc, right subclavian artery. (C) computed cardiac tomography in the axial plane in a patient with single ventricle physiology and Fontan palliation. The left pulmonary artery (LPA) is hypoplastic and required reconstruction at the time of transplantation. (D) 3D reconstruction of a cardiac computed tomography of a patient with tricuspid atresia and extracardiac Fontan. (*asterisk*) points to a large systemic venous-to-pulmonary venous collateral (*blue color*). F, extracardiac Fontan conduit. (Image courtesy of Dr. Chun (Huie) Lin.)

conditions (Fontan circulation, pulmonary atresia, and cyanosis) are thought to be potential reasons. Identification and pretransplant coiling have been proposed to decrease these bleeding complications.[15] CCT provides the highest resolution assessment for collateral vessels (**Fig. 2**D). As described in the following Fontan section, careful protocoling and imaging acquisition timing is essential to optimize diagnostic yield.

Imaging of the fontan circulation

Routine surveillance is recommended for the assessment of the long-term sequelae of Fontan palliation, such as thrombosis, right-to-left shunts, obstructive lesions, systemic AV valve dysfunction, ventricular function (systolic and diastolic), collateral burden, branch PA and Fontan obstructions and to identify complications that have prognostic implications and that might need to be addressed to optimize hemodynamics.[1] Surveillance cardiovascular testing should be performed at centers familiar with and experienced in the Fontan circulation and comfortable interpreting the results.[16] Imaging can be challenging and requires an informed understanding of the patient's anatomy and surgical history.[1] For all the modalities, a systematic approach is recommended. Patients with Fontan circulation can have a systemic left ventricle (tricuspid atresia, double inlet left ventricle, among others) or a systemic RV (hypoplastic left heart syndrome, amongst others). Some patients might have 2 good-sized ventricles, like patients with complete AV canal, in whom biventricular repair was not possible due to AV valve anatomy and technical limitations in early surgical eras.

Echocardiography It remains the first-line imaging modality for serial evaluation of patients with Fontan.[17] The current expert consensus is that these patients need a yearly echocardiogram.[16] 3D echocardiography is helpful, but large studies are required in order to assess the correlation with volumes obtained by CMR. Speckle tracking echocardiography is a reliable technique that allows for the assessment of ventricular deformation without geometric assumption and is not impacted by preload state.[18] This might provide valuable data for longitudinal follow-up, as data on prognostic value are limited.[17,19] Assessment of the presence of fenestration is particularly important in patients with cyanosis. The pressure gradient across the fenestration should be estimated with Doppler, as it reflects the transpulmonary gradient (**Fig. 3**).[17]

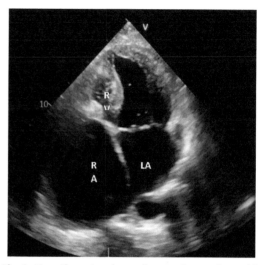

Fig. 3. Transthoracic echocardiogram in a patient with tricuspid atresia and an atrio-pulmonary (AP) Fontan.

Cardiac magnetic resonance CMR is the gold standard modality for assessing ventricular size and function. It is the current expert consensus that these patients need a CMR every 2 to 3 years, depending on their physiologic state.[1,16] CMR is effective at assessing the native anatomy, type of Fontan, patency of the Fontan pathway, presence of fenestration, branch PA stenosis, differential blood flow to the lungs, pulmonary venous anatomy, AV valve function, outflow obstruction, semilunar valve function, arch hypoplasia, or aortic coarctation. In addition, it can quantify scar and estimate collateral burden. Recent data in 416 Fontan patients suggest that increased ventricular dilatation was the strongest independent predictor of death or transplant and that associated impaired global circumferential strain identified those at the highest risk.[20]

Cardiac computed tomography In patients with Fontan circulation, imaging timing needs to be considered. A careful protocol by an experienced team is critical to optimize diagnostic yield, radiation, and contrast use. Delayed imaging to allow complete opacification of the Fontan and pulmonary arteries is vital. Different strategies can be utilized, from standardized delayed images to timing using ROI in the descending aorta or Fontan pathway to optimize imaging quality. Additional early flash acquisition might be considered to identify systemic venous to pulmonary venous collaterals from the SVC and innominate vein systems. Contrast injection side should be considered based on anatomy; sequential bilateral injections might be necessary when bilateral veno-

veno collaterals are suspected, particularly in patients with significant desaturation.

CT in patients with Fontan circulation has additional value for surgical and transplant planning, as detailed in the transplant section earlier.

Imaging of the systemic right ventricle

The RV is the systemic ventricle in patients with ccTGA and patients with D-loop TGA who have undergone the atrial switch operation (Senning or Mustard). With the transition to the arterial switch operation for patients born with D-TGA, the number of patients with a systemic RV is expected to decrease. Still, at present, it represents an important cohort of ACHD patients.[21] Systemic tricuspid regurgitation (TR) in this population represents systemic AV regurgitation, the physiologic equivalent of mitral regurgitation in a normal heart, leading to symptoms of congestive heart failure, arrhythmia, pulmonary edema, and pulmonary hypertension. In CCTA, the tricuspid valve may be congenitally abnormal, requiring surgical correction to prevent progressive systemic RV dilation and dysfunction (**Fig. 4**).[11]

Echocardiography It is considered the first-line imaging modality. The guidelines recommend these patients have a yearly echocardiogram.[1] RV ventricular assessment includes RV systolic function and RV ejection fraction, tricuspid annular plane systolic excursion, S′ velocity on tissue Doppler imaging of the tricuspid ring, and speckle tracking strain, 3D volumetric assessment from different views, including nonconventional views such as the RV inflow outflow view. The systemic tricuspid valve should be assessed in detail, including a 3D assessment. When feasible, a quantitative assessment of systemic TR should be performed. A large multicenter study of 1168 patients with D-loop TGA and atrial switch showed an association of biventricular enlargement, systolic dysfunction, and systemic TR with the primary outcome of death, transplantation, and mechanical support.[22] The value of the other parameters resides mainly in the longitudinal monitoring of each patient until more data are available. Global longitudinal and circumferential strain with CMR measured right ventricular ejection fraction has been evaluated in 2 small studies that showed conflicting data.[23,24] The correlation of subpulmonic mitral regurgitation velocity should be used to estimate left ventricle (LV) systolic pressure, which, in the absence of LV outflow tract stenosis, estimates the PA systolic pressure. Careful systemic and pulmonary venous baffle evaluation should be performed to assess for obstruction and baffle leaks in patients with atrial switch. Agitated saline contrast can be helpful when baffle leaks are suspected.

Cardiac magnetic resonance/cardiac computed tomography CMR and CCT allow precise quantification of systemic RV function via 3D reconstruction.[21] A complete assessment should also include flow acceleration with Qp: Qs calculation to assess for shunts (septal defects in ccTGA and baffle leaks in atrial switch) and branch

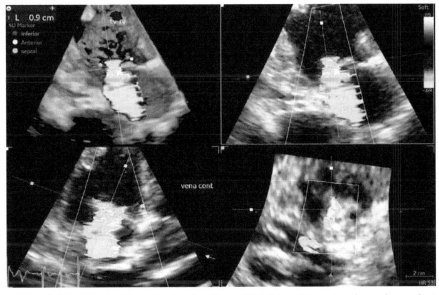

Fig. 4. Evaluation of the systemic tricuspid valve function with 3D transthoracic echocardiography in a patient with D-loop transposition of the great arteries (D-TGA) with atrial switch operation.

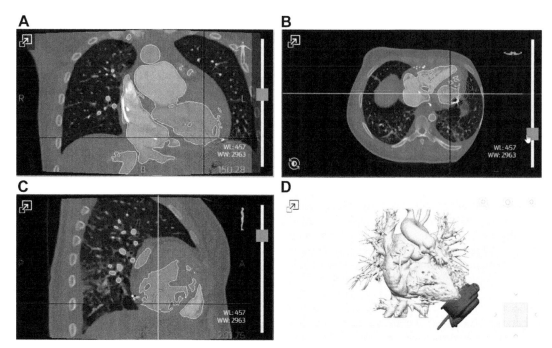

Fig. 5. Preoperative computed tomography for ventricular assist device a systemic right ventricle (sRV). Computed tomography images of a patient with congenitally corrected transposition of the great arteries with sRV (*yellow*) merged with a ventricular assist device (*red*) as part of preoperative planning. (*A*) Coronal section. (*B*) Axial section. (*C*) Sagittal section. (*D*) 3D reconstruction.

pulmonary differential flow, which can be asymmetric in cases of pulmonary venous obstructions. LGE assessment is important, as in a study of 36 patients with D-loop TGA/atrial switch, the extent of LGE correlated with ventricular dysfunction, QRS duration, and clinical events.[25] Baffle patency assessment is critical. Cine imaging of the systemic and pulmonary venous baffles can be helpful in identifying narrowing and flow acceleration. CCT may provide a more accurate assessment with less metallic artifacts in the presence of pacemaker leads or stents. In addition, CCT is useful for preoperative planning and follow-up of ventricular assist devices for the systemic RV (**Fig. 5**).

SUMMARY

The role and importance of multimodality imaging, including its applications in diagnosis, surveillance, longitudinal follow-up, and evaluation for advanced therapies in adults with CHD, are well established. It is critical that imaging in ACHD patients is performed at centers with expertise, and that the imaging protocols are tailored to the specific condition and each patient's unique native and postsurgical anatomy. Imaging in ACHD-related heart failure continues to evolve, particularly as transplant and mechanical circulatory

support are increasingly considered in this patient population. Longitudinal imaging is key for the timely identification of patients requiring evaluation for advanced therapies. Specific anatomic questions arise for preoperative planning, and multimodality imaging plays an important role in anticipating challenges and designing strategy to optimize outcomes.

CLINICS CARE POINTS

- ACHD clinical guidelines recommend routine imaging surveillance, with the frequency and modality of imaging varying according to specific conditions.

- A large multicenter study of patients with D-loop TGA and atrial switch showed an association of biventricular enlargement, systolic dysfunction, and systemic TR with the primary outcome of death, transplantation, and mechanical support.

- In a study of patients with D-loop TGA/atrial switch, the extent of LGE correlated with ventricular dysfunction, QRS duration, and clinical events.

DISCLOSURE

V.E. Duarte has no disclosures.

REFERENCES

1. Stout KK, Daniels CJ, Aboulhosn JA, et al. 2018 AHA/ACC Guideline for the Management of Adults With Congenital Heart Disease: A Report of the American College of Cardiology/American Heart Association Task Force on Clinical Practice Guidelines. Circulation 2019;139(14):e698–800.

2. Sachdeva R, Valente AM, Armstrong AK, et al. ACC/ AHA/ASE/HRS/ISACHD/SCAI/SCCT/SCMR/SOPE 2020 Appropriate Use Criteria for Multimodality Imaging During the Follow-Up Care of Patients With Congenital Heart Disease: A Report of the American College of Cardiology Solution Set Oversight Committee and Appropriate Use Criteria Task Force, American Heart Association, American Society of Echocardiography, Heart Rhythm Society, International Society for Adult Congenital Heart Disease, Society for Cardiovascular Angiography and Interventions, Society of Cardiovascular Computed Tomography, Society for Cardiovascular Magnetic Resonance, and Society of Pediatric Echocardiography. J Am Coll Cardiol 2020;75(6):657–703.

3. Zaragoza-Macias E, Schwaegler RG, Stout KK. Echocardiographic evaluation of univentricular physiology and cavopulmonary shunts. Echocardiography 2015;32(Suppl 2):S166–76.

4. Mokhles P, van den Bosch AE, Vletter-McGhie JS, et al. Feasibility and observer reproducibility of speckle tracking echocardiography in congenital heart disease patients. Echocardiography 2013; 30(8):961–6.

5. Forsey J, Friedberg MK, Mertens L. Speckle tracking echocardiography in pediatric and congenital heart disease. Echocardiography 2013;30(4): 447–59.

6. Mor-Avi V, Lang RM, Badano LP, et al. Current and evolving echocardiographic techniques for the quantitative evaluation of cardiac mechanics: ASE/ EAE consensus statement on methodology and indications endorsed by the Japanese Society of Echocardiography. Eur J Echocardiogr 2011;12(3): 167–205.

7. Bashir MR, Bhatti L, Marin D, et al. Emerging applications for ferumoxytol as a contrast agent in MRI. J Magn Reson Imag 2015;41(4):884–98.

8. Hope MD, Hope TA, Zhu C, et al. Vascular imaging with ferumoxytol as a contrast agent. AJR Am J Roentgenol 2015;205(3):W366–73.

9. Warmerdam E, Krings GJ, Leiner T, et al. Three-dimensional and four-dimensional flow assessment in congenital heart disease. Heart 2020;106(6): 421–6.

10. Bissell MM, Raimondi F, Ait Ali L, et al. 4D Flow cardiovascular magnetic resonance consensus statement: 2023 update. J Cardiovasc Magn Reson 2023;25(1):40.

11. Qureshi MY, Sommer RJ, Cabalka AK. Tricuspid valve imaging and intervention in pediatric and adult patients with congenital heart disease. JACC Cardiovasc Imaging 2019;12(4):637–51.

12. Han BK, Garcia S, Aboulhosn J, et al. Technical recommendations for computed tomography guidance of intervention in the right ventricular outflow tract: Native RVOT conduits and bioprosthetic valves:: A white paper of the Society of Cardiovascular Computed Tomography (SCCT), Congenital Heart Surgeons' Society (CHSS), and Society for Cardiovascular Angiography & Interventions (SCAI). J Cardiovasc Comput Tomogr 2023. https://doi.org/ 10.1016/j.jcct.2023.06.005 [published Online First: 20230719].

13. Rinaldi E, Sadeghi S, Rajpal S, et al. Utility of CT angiography for the prediction of coronary artery compression in patients undergoing transcatheter pulmonary valve replacement. World J Pediatr Congenit Heart Surg 2020;11(3):295–303.

14. Anwar S, Singh GK, Varughese J, et al. 3D printing in complex congenital heart disease: across a spectrum of age, pathology, and imaging techniques. JACC Cardiovasc Imaging 2017;10(8):953–6.

15. Reardon LC, DePasquale EC, Tarabay J, et al. Heart and heart-liver transplantation in adults with failing Fontan physiology. Clin Transplant 2018;32(8): e13329.

16. Rychik J, Atz AM, Celermajer DS, et al. Evaluation and management of the child and adult with fontan circulation: a scientific statement from the american heart association. Circulation 2019;140(6):e234–84 [published Online First: 20190701].

17. Moscatelli S, Borrelli N, Sabatino J, et al. Role of cardiovascular imaging in the follow-up of patients with fontan circulation. Children 2022;9(12). https://doi.org/10.3390/children9121875 [published Online First: 20221130].

18. Sutherland GR, Di Salvo G, Claus P, et al. Strain and strain rate imaging: a new clinical approach to quantifying regional myocardial function. J Am Soc Echocardiogr 2004;17(7):788–802.

19. Borrelli N, Di Salvo G, Sabatino J, et al. Serial changes in longitudinal strain are associated with outcome in children with hypoplastic left heart syndrome. Int J Cardiol 2020;317:56–62.

20. Meyer SL, St Clair N, Powell AJ, et al. Integrated clinical and magnetic resonance imaging assessments late after fontan operation. J Am Coll Cardiol 2021;77(20):2480–9.

21. Carazo M, Andrade L, Kim Y, et al. Assessment and management of heart failure in the systemic right ventricle. Heart Fail Rev 2020;25(4):609–21.

22. Broberg CS, van Dissel A, Minnier J, et al. Long-term outcomes after atrial switch operation for transposition of the great arteries. J Am Coll Cardiol 2022; 80(10):951–63.

23. Samyn MM, Yan K, Masterson C, et al. Echocardiography vs cardiac magnetic resonance imaging assessment of the systemic right ventricle for patients with d-transposition of the great arteries status post atrial switch. Congenit Heart Dis 2019;14(6): 1138–48.

24. Lipczyńska M, Szymański P, Kumor M, et al. Global longitudinal strain may identify preserved systolic function of the systemic right ventricle. Can J Cardiol 2015;31(6):760–6.

25. Babu-Narayan SV, Goktekin O, Moon JC, et al. Late gadolinium enhancement cardiovascular magnetic resonance of the systemic right ventricle in adults with previous atrial redirection surgery for transposition of the great arteries. Circulation 2005;111(16): 2091–8.

Surgical Considerations in Adult Congenital Heart Disease Heart Failure

William H. Marshall V, MD[a,b,]*, Patrick McConnell, MD[c,d]

KEYWORDS

• Fontan • Congenital heart disease • Heart failure • Transplant

KEY POINTS

• Surgical intervention is often used in the management of heart failure in patients with adult congenital heart disease to target residual lesions and valve dysfunction or pursue advanced heart failure therapies.

• There are unique anatomic and physiologic considerations for the surgeon in adults with congenital heart disease, including sternal reentry, adhesions, intracardiac and extracardiac device wires, collateral vessels, abnormal venous drainage, and the amalgamated neo-aortic root after the Damus–Kaye–Stansel procedure.

• Patient selection is of the utmost importance when considering atrioventricular valve surgery, Fontan revision, ventricular assist device, heart transplant, and combined heart–liver transplant in the management of adults with congenital heart disease and heart failure.

INTRODUCTION

Although most patients with congenital heart disease (CHD) survive into adulthood, heart failure (HF) is the leading cause of mortality in the adult CHD (ACHD) population.[1] While all patients with ACHD are at risk for HF over their lifetime, those with the highest incidence include patients with single ventricle (SV) CHD who have undergone Fontan palliation (**Fig. 1**) and those with biventricular circulation and a systemic right ventricle (sRV) (**Fig. 2**).[2] Although timing of referral for advanced HF therapies in ACHD patients is not well established, regardless of the type of CHD, surgical intervention is often used in the management of HF as care teams target residual lesions and valve dysfunction to optimize palliation, and when these strategies fail, surgery is needed for

mechanical support strategies and/or heart transplant (HT).[3] Many aspects of adults with various degrees of failed palliation over decades create unique anatomic and physiologic considerations for the surgeon. The aim of this review is to address surgical considerations in ACHD HF, discussing the role of valvular surgery and Fontan revision, as well as advanced HF therapies including ventricular assist devices (VADs) and HT (**Fig. 3**).

SURGICAL CONSIDERATIONS FOR ADULT CONGENITAL HEART DISEASE PATIENTS

Sternal Reentry

Most of the ACHD patients have prior sternotomy, and sternal reentry is often complicated by adhesions and scar tissue. This is uniquely problematic

Author Contributions: All authors contributed significantly to the concept and design, drafting, critical revision, and approval of this article.

[a] Department of Internal Medicine, Division of Cardiovascular Medicine, Davis Heart and Lung Research Institute, Wexner Medical Center at The Ohio State University, 473 West 12th Avenue Suite 200, Columbus, OH 43210, USA; [b] The Heart Center, Nationwide Children's Hospital, Columbus, OH, USA; [c] Department of Cardiothoracic Surgery, Nationwide Children's Hospital, The Heart Center, 700 Children's Drive, 4th Floor Tower, Columbus, OH 43105, USA; [d] Department of Surgery, Division of Cardiac Surgery, The Ohio State University, Columbus, OH, USA

* Corresponding author.

E-mail address: William.marshall@osumc.edu

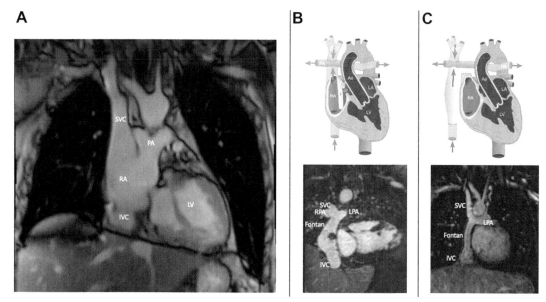

Fig. 1. Fontan types. (*A*) Cardiac magnetic resonance (CMR) image of a patient with a classic atriopulmonary Fontan. Diagram (*top*) CMR image (*bottom*) of patient with (*B*) a lateral tunnel Fontan and (*C*) an extracardiac Fontan. Ao, aorta; IVC, inferior vena cava; LA, left atrium; LPA, left pulmonary artery; LV, left ventricles; PA, pulmonary artery; RPA, right pulmonary artery; SVC, superior vena cava. (*Diagrams courtesy of* Dr Curt J. Daniels.)

in ACHD patients due to extensive mediastinal, pulmonary, and cardiac neovascularization and collateralization. In addition, known risks exist for redo-sternotomy in prior variants of dextro-transposition of the great arteries, as the neo-main pulmonary artery (after LeCompte maneuver) resides immediately below the sternum. Although likely underreported in the literature, the published incidence of major hemorrhage due to redo-sternotomy ranges from 0.6% to 6.4%, with risk of death 0.16% to 1.5% due to hemorrhage.[4] One series of 544 patients (though none with CHD) found sternal reentry injury was an independent predictor of in hospital mortality on multivariate regression.[5]

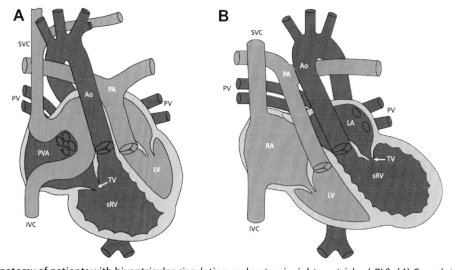

Fig. 2. Anatomy of patients with biventricular circulation and systemic right ventricles (sRV). (*A*) Complete dextro-transposition of the great arteries (concordant atrio-ventricular connection and discordant ventriculo-arterial connection) after atrial switch (Mustard or Senning) operation. (*B*) Congenitally corrected transposition of the great arteries (both discordant atrio-ventricular and ventriculo-arterial connections). Both have systemic atrioventricular valves which are morphologically tricuspid valves (TV). Ao, aorta; IVC, inferior vena cava; LA, left atrium; LV, left ventricle; PA, pulmonary artery; PV, pulmonary veins; PVA, pulmonary venous atrium; RA, right atrium; SVC, superior vena cava. (*Courtesy of* Dr Curt J. Daniels.)

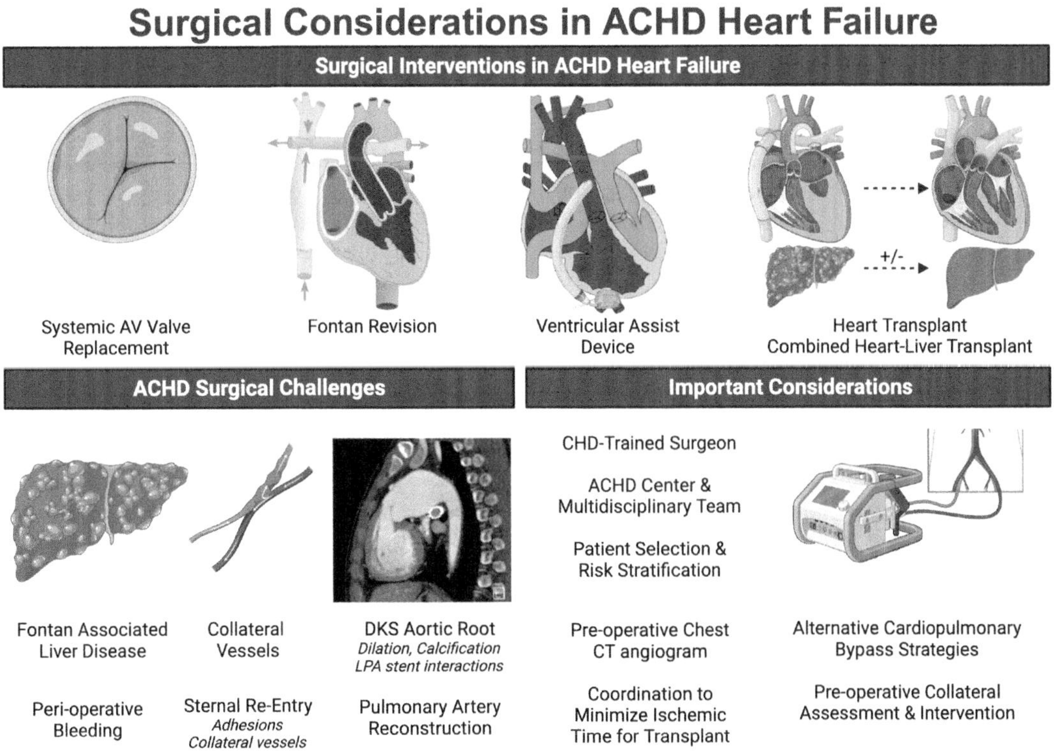

Surgical Considerations in ACHD Heart Failure

Fig. 3. Graphical abstract. ACHD, adult congenital heart disease; AV, atrioventricular; CHD, congenital heart disease; CT, computed tomography; DKS, Damus–Kaye–Stansel. (Created with BioRender.com.)

To minimize complications for redo sternotomy, a preoperative computed tomography (CT) scan can help identify high-risk anatomy, with one series reporting significantly reduced risk of sternal reentry complications in patients with versus without a preoperative CT scan.[5] Preventative strategies of sternal reentry include routine extrathoracic cardiopulmonary bypass (CPB) cannulation techniques that can mitigate some risks associated with inadvertent injuries to the heart and great vessels; in addition, many surgeons use techniques and devices to elevate the sternum and allow modest separation of tissues under the sternum before bone division. All strategies can add significant time to already complex cases, often times risking iatrogenic arryhthmias and hemodynamic instability which can be poorly tolerated, further requiring CPB be initiated from an alternative site before dissection can be completed.

Prior Cardiac Devices

A large portion of ACHD patients require pacemakers, often with multiple revisions. Therefore, transvenous and epicardial pacing or defibrillation leads may complicate the dissection or become dislodged during cardiac surgery. Although data on complications from cardiac devices during ACHD or redo surgeries are lacking, retained device components have been associated with adverse events after HT, including infectious complications.[6] Thus, balancing complete device removal while avoiding unnecessary dissection of uninvolved areas of the chest is important.

Morphologic Challenges and Considerations in Adult Congenital Heart Disease Surgical Reconstruction, Including Heart Transplant

Aortopulmonary (AP) collaterals are common in patients with a Fontan circulation (FC), though found in other ACHD patients as well, and are theorized to develop in response to chronic hypoxia. Veno-venous collaterals develop in response to higher central venous pressures within the FC and can promote progressive desaturation. Both types of collaterals can result in increased intraoperative bleeding, such that additional bypass sucker capacity is sometimes required. Moreover, higher flows on CPB are required to keep up with systemic to pulmonary artery (PA) collaterals that short circuit effective systemic circulation.[7]

Understanding the systemic venous return is paramount to safely providing effective circulatory support and assuring adequate visualization during intra-cardiac repairs. In patients with a left superior vena cava (L-SVC), direct cannulation of the L-SVC should generally be avoided, as L-SVC dissection puts the left phrenic nerve in jeopardy, and requires additional dissection leftward of either an amalgamated Damus–Kaye–Stansel (DKS) root or the main PA where the left atrial appendage or PA can be injured. Instead, strategies which avoid needless L-SVC dissection should be used. In patients with bilateral bidirectional Glenn shunts, who do not need the Fontan pathway opened, cannulating just the right SVC (toward the pulmonary caval connection) allows both SVCs to drain via the PA between the cava. In cases where the Fontan pathway is open, the surgeon may need to risk L-SVC dissection and cannulation. In regard to HT, the L-SVC should be cannulated and snared and reconstruction of the superior systemic venous anatomy should use the donor innominate vein either anterior or posterior to the aorta for reconstruction to the right atrium, in most instances via the SVC.[8]

ACHD patients undergoing HT often require reconstruction of the PAs due to branch or main PA hypoplasia, or distortion from prior shunts, Glenn, or Fontan procedures.[8] For isolated stenosis or distortion, donor and recipient PA may be adjusted as long as sufficient PA is obtained from the donor, beyond the main PA bifurcation. PA augmentation and reconstruction are specifically important for HT in patients with FC, such that some advocate for determining the need for reconstruction before HT listing,[9] with PA reconstruction performed before aortic anastomosis to allow for uninhibited access of the branch PAs.[9]

Often the most risky and difficult anatomy to contend with is the DKS root as patches used in the initial reconstruction are calcified, brittle, and intensely scared to adjacent structures (**Fig. 4**A). Heterotopic calcification often prevents the surgeon's ability to effectively or safely cross-clamp the root. Situations arise where deep hypothermic circulatory arrest is required to reconstruct the aortic arch before cross-clamping, or ventricular fibrillatory arrest is used for shorter periods where intracardiac procedures are required, though either strategy has high potential for complications. In cases of HT in patients with hypoplastic left heart syndrome, deep hypothermic circulatory arrest is increasingly required as more left PAs have been stented and thus interaction of the reconstructed aorta and the stented PA cannot be safely dissected for cross-clamping (**Fig. 4**B, C).[10] In this scenario, the branch PAs are not dissected until CPB is established to help control potentially catastrophic intraoperative bleeding.[9] However, outside of a complicated DKS root, most aortic anastomoses can be managed with adequate mobilization of the recipient's aorta and extra length of the donor aorta.[8] In patients with isolated proximal aortic arch anomalies, a hemiarch repair can be performed with an oblique anastomosis between the donor's ascending aorta and the undersurface of the recipient's aortic arch.[8]

SYSTEMIC ATRIOVENTRICULAR VALVE INTERVENTION

Valve surgery makes up the majority of surgeries performed in ACHD patients with HF. Often, valvular disease in the setting of ventricular dysfunction is amenable to surgical treatment with valve repair or replacement.[3] One population where this strategy can be successful is in patients with biventricular circulation and sRV (see **Fig. 2**) who have systemic atrioventricular valve (AVV)

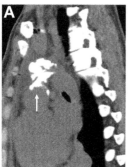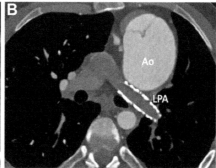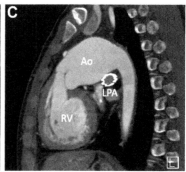

Fig. 4. Damus–Kaye–Stansel (DKS) neo-aortic root considerations. (*A*) Non-contrast computed tomography of a calcified homograft patch (*arrow*) in a patient with DKS. (*B*) Axial and (*C*) sagittal contrast-enhanced computed tomography images of a patient with DKS and neo-aortic (Ao) dilation with adjacent left pulmonary artery (LPA) stent. RV, right ventricle.

regurgitation, as they may have improvement in their functional status with tricuspid valve competency. In these patients, lower surgical mortality and morbidity is linked to preoperative sRV ejection fractions greater than 40%, particularly when AVV regurgitation represents the predominant pathology.[11] One particular difference when considering AVV surgery for ACHD patients versus adults with acquired heart disease is that tricuspid valve replacement seems more durable than repair in patients with sRVs,[12] as tricuspid valve exposure is more complicated when considering ventricular looping and position of the mass of the heart and its apex. Furthermore, many technical aspects of these complicated surgeries lead to longer aortic cross-clamp times and larger transfusion requirements which in turn have an outsized and negative impact on sRV function.

AVV regurgitation is common in patients with SV and FC, occurring in 46% to 56% of patients with common or tricuspid systemic AVV and doubling the risk of FC failure.[13] In contrast to those with biventricular circulation, the outcomes of either systemic AVV repair or replacement in patients with FC are poor, with up to 40% experiencing AVV repair failure by 3.5 years.[13] Although a consensus on timing of AVV intervention is lacking, some advocate for earlier replacement (mild-moderate regurgitation), in particular, if there is any observed decrease in systolic function.[14]

In adult patients with FC, those with the better outcomes after AVV intervention have a systemic left ventricle, with normal ventricular function.[14] Noting the multifactorial nature of AVV regurgitation in this population (abnormal leaflets, abnormal subvalvar apparatus, ventricular dilation, volume overload, and annular dilation), a combination of repair techniques including annuloplasty, cleft closure, resection, chordal transfer, "neo-chords," and Alfieri stitch may be required.[14] However, in those with systemic tricuspid valves or common AVVs, valve replacement is perhaps more appropriate, though depending on the surgical risk, evaluation for HT may be a more suitable alternative.[14] Finally, in those with severe valvular regurgitation and ventricular dysfunction, HT should be considered instead of valve surgery.[14]

All long-term data regarding the treatment of AVV regurgitation are based on surgical approaches. Interventions have begun in the catheterization laboratory with reports of transcatheter edge-to-edge repair in patients with both FC and biventricular circulation with sRVs.[15] Although surgery is avoided with its described negative impact of sRV function, the fact remains that surgical valve repair has poor outcomes beyond 1 to 2 years, and there should be little optimism for

better durability of catheter-based interventions in these anatomically complex patients. Furthermore, time and effort spent directing these complex and tenuous patients toward off-label interventions may delay, obfuscate, or prevent more timely referral for HT; thus, interventions should not be performed outside of consultation with surgeons or the HT team.

FONTAN REVISION

The original Fontan surgery was an atriopulmonary connection (see **Fig. 1**A), which over time leads to dilation of the atria and Fontan pathway. This results in an increasingly inefficient FC, further predisposing patients to atrial arrhythmias and atrial thrombus. Fontan revision requires takedown of the atriopulmonary connection, an atrial reduction plasty, atrial arrhythmia ablation, and creation of an extracardiac total cavopulmonary anastomosis. This remains a high-risk surgery with early surgical mortality as high as 12%[16] and is only advisable for teenage or younger patients with preserved ventricular systolic function who prove refractory to nonsurgical antiarrhythmic therapies. Fontan revision for patients with atriopulmonary FC has decreased significantly since 2010 as most of the patients now undergo lateral tunnel or extra-cardiac Fontan (see **Fig. 1**B, C).[17] However, enthusiasm is growing for a different type of Fontan revision that strives to ultimately increase the efficiency and loss of hemodynamic power at the cavopulmonary anastomosis by using Y-grafts to direct flow to the left and right pulmonary arteries beyond the confluence of the superior-caval connection. The rationale for pursuing and offering the Y-graft procedure is for primarily for more equitable hepatic flow to each lung and decrease pulmonary arteriovenous malformations, but also to improve the efficiency of the FC over time, as most cases have been performed within 10 years of initial Fontan procedure and not specifically for classic FC failure.[18] Given the potential morbidity and mortality from the procedure, as well as risk of further sensitization with operative exposure and transfusions, HT should also be considered if Fontan revision is being entertained as a treatment option; however, it may be a consideration in a patient with nonsurgical contraindications to transplant.

VENTRICULAR ASSIST DEVICES

Although the use of VADs in ACHD patients is increasing, this population still represents less than 1% of all VAD placements.[19] This review focuses on broad surgical considerations for the use of VADs in patients with FC and those with sRV, who present several unique challenges for surgeons as compared with the majority of patients who undergo VAD placement.

Preoperative evaluation and patient selection, specifically identifying those with appropriate hemodynamics, are key for successful VAD use in ACHD patients. Similar to patients with acquired HF, VADs can be used in patients with sRV who have developed pulmonary hypertension to improve pulmonary pressures as a potential bridge to transplant (**Fig. 5**). In patients with FC, there is still only a subset of patients with FC failure secondary to systolic dysfunction and elevated ventricular filling pressures who will receive a reliable benefit from VAD use.[20] A rather unique and key hemodynamic feature of patients particularly with FC is the presence of significant AP collaterals. These collaterals necessitate that larger flow rates are needed to satisfy systemic demands and increase the risk of vasoplegia after VAD (or HT). This is further complicated by modern durable continuous flow VADs, which are already associated with significant vasoplegia in the early post-VAD period in patients without known collaterals. Therefore, an assessment of and potential intervention on AP collaterals is needed before proceeding with VAD. Veno-venous collaterals should also be aggressively dealt with before VAD to ensure effective pulmonary blood flow after VAD.[20] The issue of Fontan fenestration closure creation at the time of VAD implant is controversial, but advocates of having an open fenestration feel that its presence assures better SV VAD filling in the acute and subacute period before the longer term salient effects of the VAD reducing transpulmonary gradients are fully realized.[20]

Many patients with either sRV or FC have had many prior operations, have residual lesions, and complex reconstructed anatomy needs to be assessed by advanced imaging with the authors favoring high-resolution CT angiogram of the whole chest, not just a cardiac CT angiogram. Not only can this define the collateral burden but also provides important information on reentry safety, concomitant, or anticipated procedures, and ultimately where the potential intracardiac and extracardiac portions of the device may be located (**Fig. 6**).[21] In addition to the previously mentioned challenges with prior DKS aortic root, this anatomy complicates where an outflow graft can safely be implanted; one alternative is sewing the outflow graft onto either the innominate or more likely the subclavian artery to avoid the DKS altogether.[20] Another consideration understands that the sRV is not a left ventricle, and thus assumptions about the structural integrity of the left ventricle do not translate to the often fat-infiltrated, thick, but structurally soft sRV-free wall. The incision in the ventricle should be at first modest and done before the cuff is sewn to the ventricle to allow enough exposure for the extensive sRV muscle bundle resection that is invariably required to avoid cannula obstruction.[20] Although the authors use three-dimensional CT simulation (see **Fig. 6**), others have reported on holographic virtual/extended reality for complex CHD VAD planning.[21]

Despite the excitement and optimism regarding VAD use in ACHD patients with HF, the morbidity burden including the risk of renal, hepatic dysfunction, and respiratory failure after VAD in ACHD patients is distinctly higher compared with patients

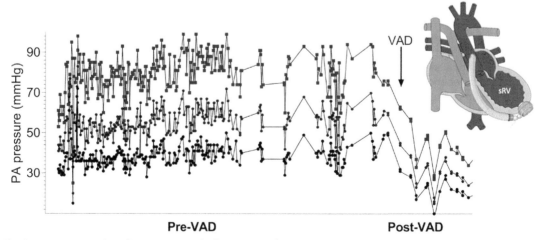

Fig. 5. Improvement in pulmonary artery (PA) pressures after ventricular assist device (VAD). PA pressures from an implanted PA pressure monitor in a patient with congenitally corrected transposition of the great arteries who underwent VAD placement in the systemic right ventricle (sRV). (Created with BioRender.com).

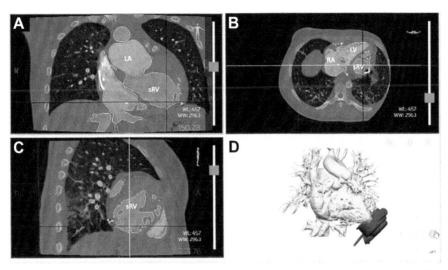

Fig. 6. Preoperative computed tomography for ventricular assist device a systemic right ventricle (sRV). Computed tomography images of a patient with congenitally corrected transposition of the great arteries with sRV (*yellow*) merged with a ventricular assist device (*red*) as part of preoperative planning. (*A*) Coronal section, (*B*) axial section, (*C*) sagittal section, and (*D*) 3D reconstruction. LA, left atrium; LV, left ventricle; RA, right atrium.

with non-ACHD HF.[19] Furthermore, in this population with already potentially high allosensitization, surgery for VAD placement can increase antibody formation,[22] which must be considered in the overall treatment strategy. Thus, HT remains the main surgical procedure for end-stage HF in ACHD patients.

ADULT CONGENITAL HEART DISEASE HEART TRANSPLANT
Surgical Risk

Before imparting on a discussion of surgical technique for HT in ACHD patients, a brief mention of surgical risk stratification is important, including

Table 1
Risk score of adult congenital orthotopic heart transplant

Risk Factor	Points Assigned
Patient age <30 y	0
Patient age ≥ 30 y	2
Dialysis-dependent	4
Ventilator-dependent	4
Serum total bilirubin ≥ 2.4 mg/dL	3
Total potential points	13

Score developed by Seese L, Morell VO, Viegas M, et al. A Risk Score for Adults With Congenital Heart Disease Undergoing Heart Transplantation. *The Annals of Thoracic Surgery.* 2021;111(6):2033-2040.

operator and institutional variables. It is noteworthy that overall surgical outcomes are better for ACHD patients with a surgeon trained in CHD[23] with some evidence supporting HT outcomes in ACHD patients are improved with a CHD surgeon.[24] Similarly, ACHD patients have better outcomes when undergoing HT at accredited ACHD centers and centers that perform higher volume of CHD transplants.[25,26] Therefore, center volume, institutional experience, and CHD surgical expertise are all essential when considering HT in ACHD patients.

In terms of predicting surgical risk, one study using United Network for Organ Sharing data developed a 13-point risk score for ACHD patients undergoing HT (**Table 1**).[27] In patients with 4 or more points, posttransplant mortality, renal failure requiring dialysis, and median length of hospital stay were all higher.[27] It is important to note a limitation of this study is the inability to discern type of CHD; thus, it is unclear how the above risk score (see **Table 1**)[27] differs for patients with FC as compared with those with biventricular CHD. Although not a surgical risk calculator, in a group of patients with FC, posttransplant outcomes were worse in patients with increased time from the Fontan to transplant evaluation, the New York Heart Association class IV functional status, lower extremity varicosities, and increased veno-venous collaterals.[28] One study has reported on the use of deep machine learning to predict transplant surgical risk in SV patients[29]; thus, further innovations are sure to develop with the increasing use of artificial intelligence in CHD.[30]

Fontan-Specific Heart Transplant Considerations

In addition to redo sternotomy, sensitization from prior surgeries and other complications common to all ACHD patients with HF, there are some risks that are more prevalent (though not exclusive) in patients with FC, including collateral vessels and liver disease, both of which contribute to perioperative bleeding risk.31

Management of collateral vessels is important in the planning for HT, as intraoperative hemorrhage was identified as a significant risk factor for early mortality in a cohort of 31 patients with FC.[31] Many centers advocate for periodic collateral occlusion, some as often as every 3 months while listed for transplant.[32]

Another consideration in the evaluation for potential HT perioperative morbidity in patients with FC is an assessment of liver function, as Fontan-associated liver disease (FALD) is almost universal within 20 years of initial Fontan surgery.[33] In patients with non-congenital HF, the presence of advanced liver disease and cirrhosis is contradictions to isolated HT due to unacceptably high short-term mortality.[34] However, despite the high prevalence of FALD, not all patients with FC require combined heart–liver transplant (CHLT). The authors believe one reason may be that in cases of acquired HF associated with liver failure, the aggravating features to the liver disease are often noncardiac; thus, transplant does not singularly fix all insults, is associated with more advanced age of the patient, and typically impacts liver synthetic function more dramatically than is typically encountered in FALD. Therefore, the treating multidisciplinary HT team must understand FALD as a separate entity.

The evaluation of liver disease for patients under consideration for HT is beyond the scope of this article. Briefly, recent consensus guidelines recommend HT alone can be considered in those with elevated model for end-stage liver disease-excluding international normalized ratio score, ascites, or thrombocytopenia if there is no cirrhosis on biopsy and the hepatic wedge pressure is low.[34] Thus, there may be benefit of CHLT in a subset of patients with advanced liver disease, though there is still no uniform recommendation for which patients with FC should undergo HT versus CHLT.

CHLT can be performed either sequentially or en bloc, with center-specific preference for these techniques.[34] For sequential CHLT, after the HT is performed, the aortic cross-clamp is removed allowing for reperfusion of the heart and the liver transplant can then commence. In some cases, the patient may be maintained on CPB, in others it may be weaned, and the chest is left open during the liver transplant.[35] In the en bloc technique, during procurement, the cardiac surgeons perform the midline sternotomy which is extended below the umbilicus by the liver surgeons, and after dissection and aortic cross-clamp, the organs are removed and packaged together.[36] In the recipient, after CBP, hepatectomy and cardiectomy, the heart–liver graft is placed starting with the left atrial anastomosis and the two teams work simultaneously to complete the cardiac and hepatic vascular anastomoses. After the heart is adequately re-perfused and both organs are in optimal condition, CBP is removed and the liver surgeons complete the biliary anastomosis.[36]

Ischemic Time

Owing to the described operative complexity, ischemic time is longer in HT for patients with FC, which is a known risk factor for posttransplant mortality. Therefore, meticulous coordination between the procuring and transplant teams is required to minimize ischemic time and improve outcomes. It is critical to perform the reconstruction of the anastomotic sites before arrival of the donor heart, and some advocate for allowing at least 4 hours for the dissection and reconstruction.[37] The systemic venous reconstruction can be achieved using donor innominate vein in most cases, and although some prefer donor tissue for PA and aortic reconstruction,[7] others advocate for using homograft or prosthetic material and not waiting for donor material given the time required for these procedures.[37]

Postoperative Considerations

There is a high incidence of postoperative graft failure in patients with FC after HT.[9] Owing to the denervated state of the heart, extra inotropic support while maintaining a high heart rate as well as pulmonary vasodilators is needed to successfully wean from bypass. Failure is often attributed to the right ventricle, but high AP collateral flow requires even the left ventricle to take on supraphysiologic loads in the early postoperative period, further aggravating states of hypotension and vasoplegia. Thus, vasopressors should be readily used, with a low threshold for extracorporeal life support to provide the high outputs that the heart graft cannot support in the early hours after HT in many patients with significant collaterals.

SUMMARY

In summary, HF is a common complication in patients with ACHD which often requires surgical intervention. Although VAD and HT are options for late-stage HF in the ACHD patient, redo-sternotomy, bleeding risk, and end-organ dysfunction offer significant surgical risks which must be mitigated. Nevertheless, successful surgical intervention is possible in this complex population of patients with a CHD-trained surgeon, appropriate risk stratification, and meticulous surgical planning.

CLINICS CARE POINTS

- Unique surgical considerations in adults with congenital heart disease (ACHD) include sternal reentry, adhesions, intracardiac and extracardiac device wires, collateral vessels, abnormal venous drainage, and the dilated and/or calcified neo-aortic root after the Damus–Kaye–Stansel procedure.

- Understanding the systemic venous return is paramount to safely providing effective circulatory support and assuring adequate visualization during intra-cardiac repairs in ACHD patients.

- Systemic atrioventricular valve surgery in adults with biventricular congenital heart disease and systemic right ventricles can improve functional status with better outcomes performed before the onset of significant ventricular dysfunction.

- The subset of patients for which Fontan revision is appropriate is limited.

- Ventricular assist devices are feasible in ACHD patients with appropriate patient selection and preoperative CT imaging, though the risk of end-organ dysfunction is higher than in patients with non-ACHD heart failure.

- Collateral vessel assessment and intervention should be performed for patients with a Fontan circulation undergoing ventricular assist device placement or heart transplant.

- Outcomes for heart transplant in ACHD patients are improved with a congenital heart disease-trained surgeon, at ACHD-accredited programs, with higher ACHD transplant volumes.

- Combined heart–liver transplant is appropriate for a subset of patients with a Fontan circulation and can be performed sequentially or *en bloc*, with center-specific preference for these techniques

DISCLOSURE

All authors have reported that they have no relationships relevant to the contents of this article to disclose. No artificial intelligence software was used in the development of this article.

REFERENCES

1. Diller GP, Kempny A, Alonso-Gonzalez R, et al. Survival Prospects and Circumstances of Death in Contemporary Adult Congenital Heart Disease Patients Under Follow-Up at a Large Tertiary Centre. Circulation 2015;132(22):2118–25.
2. Bruaene AVD, Hickey EJ, Kovacs AH, et al. Phenotype, management and predictors of outcome in a large cohort of adult congenital heart disease patients with heart failure. Int J Cardiol 2018;252:80–7.
3. Hörer J. Current spectrum, challenges and new developments in the surgical care of adults with congenital heart disease. Cardiovasc Diagn Ther 2018;8(6):754–64.
4. Morales D, Williams E, John R. Is resternotomy in cardiac surgery still a problem? Interact Cardiovasc Thorac Surg 2010;11(3):277–86.
5. Imran Hamid U, Digney R, Soo L, et al. Incidence and outcome of re-entry injury in redo cardiac surgery: benefits of preoperative planning. Eur J Cardio Thorac Surg 2015;47(5):819–23.
6. Fardman A, Ram E, Lavee J, et al. Complications of retained pacemaker hardware in heart transplant recipients: case series and review of the literature. Infection 2020;48(4):635–40.
7. Mauchley DC, Mitchell MB. Transplantation in the Fontan Patient. Semin Thorac Cardiovasc Surg Pediatr Card Surg Annu 2015;18(1):7–16.
8. Hosseinpour AR, González-Calle A, Adsuar-Gómez A, et al. Surgical technique for heart transplantation: a strategy for congenital heart disease. Eur J Cardio Thorac Surg 2013;44(4):598–604.
9. Bryant R, Morales D. Overview of adult congenital heart transplants. Ann Cardiothorac Surg 2018; 7(1):143–51.
10. Iyengar AJ, Sharma VJ, d'Udekem Y, et al. Aortic arch and pulmonary artery reconstruction during heart transplantation after failed Fontan procedure. Interact Cardiovasc Thorac Surg 2014;18(5):693–4.
11. Mongeon FP, Connolly HM, Dearani JA, et al. Congenitally corrected transposition of the great arteries ventricular function at the time of systemic atrioventricular valve replacement predicts long-term ventricular function. J Am Coll Cardiol 2011; 57(20):2008–17.
12. Koolbergen DR, Ahmed Y, Bouma BJ, et al. Follow-up after tricuspid valve surgery in adult patients with systemic right ventricles. Eur J Cardio Thorac Surg 2016;50(3):456–63.

13. King G, Ayer J, Celermajer D, et al. Atrioventricular Valve Failure in Fontan Palliation. J Am Coll Cardiol 2019;73(7):810–22.

14. Stephens EH, Dearani JA. Management of the bad atrioventricular valve in Fontan… time for a change. J Thorac Cardiovasc Surg 2019;158(6):1643–8.

15. Silini A, Iriart X. Percutaneous edge-to-edge repair in congenital heart disease: Preliminary results of a promising new technique. International Journal of Cardiology Congenital Heart Disease 2022;8: 100370.

16. Jacobs JP, Maruszewski B. Functionally univentricular heart and the fontan operation: lessons learned about patterns of practice and outcomes from the congenital heart surgery databases of the European association for cardio-thoracic surgery and the society of thoracic surgeons. World J Pediatr Congenit Heart Surg 2013;4(4):349–55.

17. Backer CL, Mavroudis C. 149 Fontan Conversions. Methodist Debakey Cardiovasc J 2019;15(2): 105–10.

18. Trusty PM, Wei Z, Sales M, et al. Y-graft modification to the Fontan procedure: Increasingly balanced flow over time. J Thorac Cardiovasc Surg 2020;159(2): 652–61.

19. VanderPluym CJ, Cedars A, Eghtesady P, et al. Outcomes following implantation of mechanical circulatory support in adults with congenital heart disease: An analysis of the Interagency Registry for Mechanically Assisted Circulatory Support (INTERMACS). J Heart Lung Transplant 2018;37(1):89–99.

20. Villa C, Greenberg JW, Morales DLS. Mechanical support for the failing single ventricle after Fontan. JTCVS Tech 2022;13:174–81.

21. Szugye NA, Zafar F, Villa C, et al. 3D Holographic Virtual Surgical Planning for a Single Right Ventricle Fontan Patient Needing Heartmate III Placement. ASAIO J 2021;67(12):e211–5.

22. Kwon MH, Zhang JQ, Schaenman JM, et al. Characterization of ventricular assist device-mediated sensitization in the bridge-to-heart-transplantation patient. J Thorac Cardiovasc Surg 2015;149(4): 1161–6.

23. Karamlou T, Diggs BS, Person T, et al. National Practice Patterns for Management of Adult Congenital Heart Disease. Circulation 2008;118(23):2345–52.

24. Mori M, Vega D, Book W, et al. Heart Transplantation in Adults With Congenital Heart Disease: 100% Survival With Operations Performed by a Surgeon Specializing in Congenital Heart Disease in an Adult Hospital. Ann Thorac Surg 2015;99(6):2173–8.

25. Nguyen VP, Dolgner SJ, Dardas TF, et al. Improved Outcomes of Heart Transplantation in Adults With Congenital Heart Disease Receiving Regionalized Care. J Am Coll Cardiol 2019;74(23):2908–18.

26. Menachem JN, Lindenfeld J, Schlendorf K, et al. Center volume and post-transplant survival among adults with congenital heart disease. J Heart Lung Transplant 2018;37(11):1351–60.

27. Seese L, Morell VO, Viegas M, et al. A Risk Score for Adults With Congenital Heart Disease Undergoing Heart Transplantation. Ann Thorac Surg 2021; 111(6):2033–40.

28. Lewis MJ, Reardon LC, Aboulhosn J, et al. Morbidity and Mortality in Adult Fontan Patients After Heart or Combined Heart-Liver Transplantation. J Am Coll Cardiol 2023;81(22):2161–71.

29. Jalali A, Lonsdale H, Do N, et al. Deep Learning for Improved Risk Prediction in Surgical Outcomes. Sci Rep 2020;10(1):9289.

30. Jone PN, Gearhart A, Lei H, et al. Artificial Intelligence in Congenital Heart Disease. JACC (J Am Coll Cardiol): Advances 2022;1(5):100153.

31. Cardoso B, Kelecsenyi A, Smith J, et al. Improving outcomes for transplantation in failing Fontan— what is the next target? JTCVS Open 2021;8: 565–73.

32. Tan W, Reardon L, Lin J, et al. Occlusion of aortopulmonary and venovenous collaterals prior to heart or combined heart-liver transplantation in Fontan patients: A single-center experience. International Journal of Cardiology Congenital Heart Disease 2021;6:100260.

33. Munsterman ID, Duijnhouwer AL, Kendall TJ, et al. The clinical spectrum of Fontan-associated liver disease: results from a prospective multimodality screening cohort. Eur Heart J 2019;40(13):1057–68.

34. Kittleson MM, Sharma KS, Brennan DC, et al. Dual-Organ Transplantation: Indications, Evaluation, and Outcomes for Heart-Kidney and Heart-Liver Transplantation: A Scientific Statement From the American Heart Association. Circulation 2023. https://doi.org/10.1161/CIR.0000000000001155.

35. Reardon LC, DePasquale EC, Tarabay J, et al. Heart and heart–liver transplantation in adults with failing Fontan physiology. Clin Transplant 2018;32(8): e13329.

36. Vaikunth SS, Concepcion W, Daugherty T, et al. Short-term outcomes of en bloc combined heart and liver transplantation in the failing Fontan. Clin Transplant 2019;33(6):e13540.

37. Konstantinov IE, Schulz A, Buratto E. Heart transplantation after Fontan operation. JTCVS Tech 2022;13:182–91.

Pulmonary Hypertension in Adult Congenital Heart Disease–Related Heart Failure

Jonathan Kusner, MD[a], Richard A. Krasuski, MD[b],*

KEYWORDS

- Congenital • Heart disease • Pulmonary hypertension • Vasodilator • Heart failure
- Pulmonary vascular resistance

KEY POINTS

- Elevated pulmonary vascular resistance (PVR) in the setting of adult congenital heart disease (ACHD) complicated by heart failure (HF) requires careful assessment of pulmonary and systemic flows.
- In the setting of HF, the initiation of pulmonary vasodilators can only occur safely in a closely monitored setting.
- Managing elevated PVRs in the setting of ACHD-HF uses medical, interventional, and surgical techniques that must be considered by a multidisciplinary management team.

INTRODUCTION

The longer life expectancies for individuals with congenital heart disease (CHD) are a testament to dramatic advances in care and collaboration across the medical, interventional, and surgical care continua. Life spans have steadily lengthened, with contemporary estimates of median survival for those with simple lesions at more than 60 years and more than 30 years for those with the most complex of lesions.[1,2] As these individuals age into adulthood, they encounter diseases of adulthood, most notably heart failure (HF), which remains a major driver of morbidity and mortality in the adult congenital heart disease (ACHD) population.[3]

ACHD-related HF (ACHD-HF) remains a heterogeneous set of conditions without a consensus definition. These disease processes are diverse and, in contrast to non-CHD-related HF, rarely have a precipitating event that incites adverse remodeling, neurohormonal changes, and clinical decompensation. Instead, many of these individuals have never had a normal myocardium and remain vulnerable to the insidious onset of ventricular dysfunction, a process only hastened by traditional vascular risk factors encountered in adulthood. Given this, early and aggressive cardiovascular risk factor modification remains a cornerstone of management.[4]

One additional element that dramatically complicates the management of ACHD-HF is the development of elevated pulmonary vascular resistance (PVR). For the broad population of ACHD, a diagnosis of pulmonary hypertension (PH) is associated with a two-fold higher risk of all-cause mortality and a three-fold higher rate of health care utilization, reflecting considerably higher morbidity.[5] Patients with ACHD-HF will often develop elevated pulmonary pressures related to their elevated systemic ventricular filling pressures. This review instead focuses on conditions whereby these elevations are disproportionate to systemic filling pressures, that is, elevated PVR. The classification of PH and ACHD-related pulmonary arterial hypertension

[a] Department of Medicine, Duke University Medical Center, 2301 Erwin Road, Durham, NC 27705, USA;
[b] Department of Cardiovascular Medicine, Duke University Medical Center, Box 3012, Durham, NC 27710, USA
* Corresponding author.
E-mail address: richard.krasuski@duke.edu

Heart Failure Clin 20 (2024) 209–221
https://doi.org/10.1016/j.hfc.2023.12.010
1551-7136/24/© 2023 Elsevier Inc. All rights reserved.

(PAH) is reviewed, followed by a discussion of specific management considerations when treating HF in patients with ACHD with elevated PVR.

PULMONARY HYPERTENSION CLASSIFICATION

Convened in 2019, the 6th World Symposium on Pulmonary Hypertension revised existing hemodynamic thresholds to redefine PH as a mean pulmonary artery pressure (mPAP) greater than 20 mm Hg.[6] Many disparate disease processes elevate mPAP beyond this threshold; these conditions have been categorized into 5 groups (**Table 1**). Consistent with the heterogeneity of CHD, patients with ACHD encounter PH related to causes that span all 5 categories and often experience pathophysiologies that overlap multiple existing groupings.

Group 1 Pulmonary Hypertension

PAH, also known as Group 1 PH, describes PH in which elevations in mPAP greater than 20 mm Hg occur in the setting of pulmonary capillary wedge pressure (PCWP) $\leq$ 15 mm Hg and a PVR $\geq$ 2 Wood units (WU).[7]

Many CHD lesions predispose to the development of PAH through the presence of systemic-to-pulmonary shunts that lead to volume, and in some instances pressure, overload of the pulmonary circulation (**Table 2**). In this setting, the development of PAH appears to be defect dependent, with ventricular septal defect (VSD), atrial septal defect (ASD), and persistent ductus arteriosus (PDA) being the most common, and may have contributions from environmental, genetic, and epigenetic factors.[8,9]

Increases in pulmonary blood flow (Qp) instigate multifactorial mechanisms, including increased sheer stress, endothelial damage, changes in vasoactive mediators and growth factors, that contribute to vasoconstriction, further endothelial dysfunction, neomuscularization, proliferative and obstructive remodeling, inflammation, and thrombosis that serve to elevate mPAP.[10–14] These mechanisms are similar to other forms of PAH and are characterized cellularly by dysregulation of proliferative and apoptotic factors. Although initially reversible and occurring at points of perturbed blood flow, particularly at distal pulmonary arterial branch points, if untreated this process can progress to irreversible stages, characterized by general neointimal fibrosis and the formation of plexus channels (**Fig. 1**).[11,15] Although patients with ACHD most commonly encounter these changes in the setting of volume overload, pressure overload further compounds these processes; individuals with pre-tricuspid valve (TV)

Table 1 Classification of pulmonary hypertension according to the 6th World Symposium on Pulmonary Hypertension	
Pulmonary Hypertension Classification	
Group	Cause
Group 1	**PAH** CHD Idiopathic Heritable Drug or toxin induced Persistent PH of the newborn Pulmonary veno-occlusive disease Connective tissue diseases Human immunodeficiency virus infection Portal hypertension Schistosomiasis Chronic hemolytic anemia
Group 2	**PH caused by left heart disease** Systolic dysfunction Diastolic dysfunction Valvular heart disease
Group 3	**PH caused by lung disease or hypoxia** Chronic obstructive lung disease Interstitial lung disease Mixed restrictive/obstructive lung disease Sleep-disordered breathing Chronic exposure to high altitude
Group 4	**Chronic thromboembolic PH**
Group 5	**PH with unclear or multifactorial mechanisms** Hematologic disorders Myeloproliferative disorders Splenectomy Systemic disorders Sarcoidosis Langerhans cell histiocytosis Metabolic disorders Glycogen storage disease Gaucher disease Thyroid disorders Others Tumoral obstruction Fibrosing mediastinitis Chronic renal failure on dialysis

Table 2
Clinical classification of pulmonary arterial hypertension in congenital heart disease

Eisenmenger syndrome	Large left-to-right shunt that leads to severe elevation in PVR and shunt reversal Characterized by hypoxia and central cyanosis
Persistent left-to-right shunt	Moderate to large left-to-right shunt resulting in increased PVR May or may not be correctable May or may not be reversible
Coincidental CHD	Elevation of PVR is out of proportion to the magnitude of shunt and the size of the congenital heart lesion The congenital heart defect is unlikely to be directly responsible for the development of PAH
Postinterventional	PAH that either persists after shunt closure or develops months or years after index intervention
Other	Segmental PAH. This can be related to pulmonary atresia or altered pulmonary arterial flow conditions that were present during development or acquired later in life

lesions, characterized by low pressure left-to-right or bidirectional shunts that lead to elevated Qp, do not uniformly develop ACHD-PAH. If they do develop PAH, disease onset tends to be well into the fourth decade of life.[16] This is in contrast to post-TV lesions that, depending on lesion size, are characterized by high-pressure left-to-right shunts that expose the pulmonary vasculature to pressure and volume overload, often leading to PAH within the first years of life if unrepaired.[17,18]

Group 2 Pulmonary Hypertension

Throughout this review, for individuals with ACHD with 2 ventricles, the term subpulmonary ventricle will be used in reference to the ventricle supplying blood to the pulmonary vascular beds, and the term systemic ventricle will be used to signify to the ventricle supplying blood to the rest of the body. The terms left and right will refer to the morphologic left and right ventricles, respectively, regardless of anatomic positioning. Group 2 PH refers to disease caused by cardiac dysfunction. Most commonly this is related to systemic ventricular dysfunction, but can also occur related to systemic valvular lesions or obstructive aortic pathologic conditions resulting in elevated filling diastolic filling pressures that are transmitted through the pulmonary vasculature, ultimately elevating mPAP. In this condition, PCWP is greater than 15 mm Hg, although PVR is often low, less than 2 WU.[19]

Importantly, patients with Group 2 PH may develop mixed disease in which PCWP is greater than 15 mm Hg along with mPAP that is elevated disproportionately, and thus elevated PVR. Management considerations of this condition will be discussed further.

Group 3 Pulmonary Hypertension

PH caused by lung disease is referred to as Group 3 disease. This includes any obstructive or restrictive processes that may contribute to prolonged hypoxic vasoconstriction or other pulmonary remodeling that may elevate mPAP.[20] In the ACHD population, individuals often have experienced multiple sternotomies or thoracotomies by adulthood, resulting in restrictive chest wall disease and inefficient ventilation, the end result of which can be PH.

Group 4 Pulmonary Hypertension

Group 4 PH is related to chronic pulmonary artery (PA) obstruction. This includes chronic thromboembolic pulmonary hypertension (CTEPH), although, importantly, is broadened in recent guidelines to include congenital lesions (ie, branch PA stenosis) in addition to acquired obstruction.[7] In all patient groups, Group 4 PH is often underrecognized and associated with high morbidity and mortality.[21] Patients with ACHD face particular challenges; they may experience comorbid thromboembolic disease leading to CTEPH, and diagnosis can be further complicated by misattribution of clinical findings; for example, large bronchial artery collaterals typically elevate concern for CTEPH, although in the ACHD population these may be incorrectly construed as part of an individual's CHD.[22,23]

Group 5 Pulmonary Hypertension

Group 5 PH is disease related to multifactorial mechanisms, often associated with systemic processes. The most complex forms of CHD-PAH have been classified as Group 5 disease.

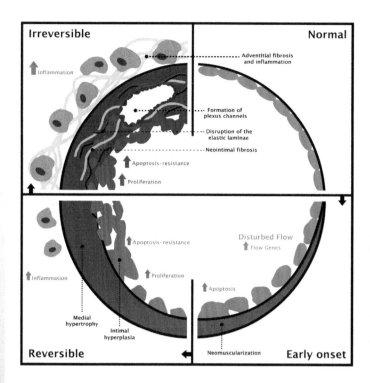

Fig. 1. Many CHD lesions predispose to the development of PAH through the presence of systemic-to-pulmonary shunts that lead to volume, and in some instances pressure, overload of the pulmonary circulation. Increases in Qp instigate multifactorial mechanisms, including increased sheer stress, endothelial damage, changes in vasoactive mediators and growth factors, that contribute to vasoconstriction, further endothelial dysfunction, neomuscularization, proliferative and obstructive remodeling, inflammation, and thrombosis that serve to elevate mPAP. These mechanisms are similar to other forms of PAH and are characterized cellularly by dysregulation of proliferative and apoptotic factors. Although initially reversible and occurring at points of perturbed blood flow, if untreated, this process can progress to irreversible stages, characterized by general neointimal fibrosis and the formation of plexus channels.

CLASSIFICATION OF ADULT CONGENITAL HEART DISEASE–RELATED PULMONARY ARTERIAL HYPERTENSION

For individuals with CHD in the neonatal and pediatric intervals, clinicians must remain mindful of the relative blood flow through the pulmonary and systemic capillary beds (Qp:Qs). This ratio is typically 1:1, indicating that no net shunting is occurring. Attention to this value is needed in CHD given the variety of lesions that may allow for intracardiac or extracardiac shunting and given the importance of balancing these flows; too little Qp impairs proper pulmonary vascular development, whereas too much Qp can promote adverse vascular remodeling.[24–26] Given the many conditions that lead to ACHD-PAH, a clinical classification system has been developed that should be considered whenever interrogating Group 1 causes of elevated PVRs in the setting of ACHD-HF, given that identification of distinct entities within this classification scheme may provide a path forward for further diagnosis and management. The 5 clinical subgroups include Eisenmenger syndrome (ES), PAH associated with persistent systemic-to-pulmonary shunts, PAH with small or coincidental shunts, PAH with persistent shunts or those that develop following repair, and segmental PAH.

Eisenmenger Syndrome

Dr Victor Eisenmenger in 1897 described what is now known as Eisenmenger syndrome, the severest form of ACHD PAH. ES represents pathologic adaptation to persistent left-to-right shunting with resulting "pulmonary hypertension due to high pulmonary vascular resistance with reversed or bidirectional shunt at the aortopulmonary, ventricular, or atrial level," as articulated in 1958 by Dr Paul Wood.[27] It occurs most often related to lesions that promote persistent pulmonary overcirculation in which the subpulmonic ventricle experiences persistent pressure and volume overload.[28,29]

Pulmonary Arterial Hypertension Associated with Persistent Systemic-to-Pulmonary Shunts

Patients with significant and persistent systemic-to-pulmonary shunts do not uniformly progress to ES. Many of these patients develop PAH with mildly to moderately elevated PVR, an insufficient level to precipitate shunt reversal. Here, cyanosis is not present at rest, although could develop in situations when PVR acute increases or systemic vascular resistance drops, like during or following heavy exertion. Early identification and assessment of Qp:Qs in these individuals is important, as timely shunt closure may halt or reverse progression of pulmonary vascular disease. In the context of ACHD-HF, this category must be considered carefully, as interventions aimed at improving cardiac output (ie, pharmacologic afterload reduction) can impact shunting.

Pulmonary Arterial Hypertension with Coincidental Shunts

This category describes patients that have elevated PVR in whom small and unrelated shunts have been discovered. In such cases, these very small shunts are unlikely to be driving elevated PVR, and additional diagnostic testing should be pursued to identify additional causes of PAH or other groups of PH that may be concomitant. These individuals appear to have a similar prognosis to idiopathic PAH.[30] Closures (surgical or transcatheter) for these coincidental shunts may have detrimental effects and are generally ill-advised.

Pulmonary Arterial Hypertension After Defect Closure

Patients with PAH after defect closure consist of the 2 following groups: those who develop PAH years after defect closure and those who experience persistent PAH following defect closure. These 2 forms have been shown to occur in ~3% of patients following defect repair.[31] The driving factors for the later development of PAH in the former group are not well understood, although persistent atrial fibrillation following ASD correction has been associated with this phenotype.[32] The latter group consists generally of shunts diagnosed later in life for whom closure alone no longer significantly modifies the disease process. Several clinical characteristics help to identify patients most likely to encounter persistently elevated PVR following closure, including older age at repair, female sex, large defect size, complete atrioventricular septal defect and sinus venosus defect, Qp:Qs $\geq$ 3, pulmonary systolic pressure greater than 40 mm Hg before closure, and the presence of an associated genetic syndrome.[33] Even outside of the context of HF, this form of ACHD-PAH has a particularly poor prognosis.[31,34]

Segmental Pulmonary Arterial Hypertension

This form of PH refers to nonuniform remodeling of the pulmonary vasculature in a manner whereby discrete sections of the lung have elevated PVR, whereas other segments have comparatively lower or near normal PVR. The development of segmental PAH is related to flow perturbations that disproportionately deliver blood to specific pulmonary vascular beds. This may occur in the setting of congenital or acquired causes, including peripheral PA stenosis; single, absent, or atretic PA; anomalous PA feeding a single lung segment; and following ineffective PA banding or surgical shunts (ie, Potts and Waterston).

DIAGNOSTIC CONSIDERATIONS
Transthoracic Echocardiogram

Transthoracic echocardiography (TTE) is one of the critical first steps in the evaluation of patients with ACHD with HF suspected to have elevated PVR. It should ideally be performed by a sonographer with experience in imaging adults with CHD and interpreted by an ACHD board-certified cardiologist. From TTE, the tricuspid regurgitant velocity is estimated to further elevate suspicion for PH.[7,35,36]

TTE is also crucial in the assessment of ventricular function. Any increase in subpulmonic ventricular internal dimensions or reduction in systolic function should increase suspicion for the underlying presence of PAH. TTE is also useful to identify and characterize intracardiac or aortopulmonary shunts or evidence of incomplete or failed correction. Shunt fractions can change in the setting of HF or changes in PVR and should be recharacterized by TTE. Qp:Qs can be noninvasively calculated using Doppler imaging, and contrast (bubble) study can identify abnormal mixing of circulations. These communications can place abnormal stress on one or both ventricles and contribute to acute clinical decompensation.

Cardiac Magnetic Resonance Imaging

Cardiac MRI can be useful to further characterize the location and size of shunting. This modality can help further delineate the degree of shunting and facilitate anatomic measurements to determine feasibility and probability of successful defect closure.

Heart Catheterization

Right heart catheterization (RHC) represents the gold standard for diagnosing PH. RHC has great utility when there is concern for elevated PVR in the setting of AHCD-HF, given that it can measure PVR directly and parse overlapping drivers of PH. Specifically, for patients with HF, RHC can determine whether PH elevations are purely related to elevations in left atrial pressure or whether there may be mixed disease in which elevation in PVR is also present.[19] The operator must be meticulous in data collection to ensure that subsequent calculations are accurate. Oxygen saturations must be collected before the location of the shunt to appropriately delineate the step-up in saturation and thus the Qp:Qs and PVR. Anomalous pulmonary veins can be present in ~10% of patients with ASDs and are universally present in sinus venosus defects. For this reason, collection of a "high" superior vena cava saturation is crucial. In some patients with longstanding PH, the pulmonary arteries can be dilated and tortuous, making wedge pressure determination challenging. Although measuring left ventricular end-diastolic pressure would be standard practice under such circumstances, this can potentially miss a stiff left atrium (as can be seen in some patients with HF with preserved systolic function) or pulmonary venous stenosis (as can be present owing to CHD or as a result of prior pulmonary vein isolation for atrial fibrillation). Invasive hemodynamics are strongly recommended before the initiation of any targeted PAH therapies or defect closure. For some patients, invasive measures of hemodynamics during exercise can help to distinguish between left heart and right heart predominant lesions. Patients can also undergo a "vasodilator challenge" with careful observation of PA and PCWP to assess the hemodynamic response. Finally, the defect can be transiently occluded with a balloon and hemodynamics remeasured to ensure that this is well tolerated before an occluder device is implanted or surgical repair is performed.

MANAGEMENT CONSIDERATIONS

For patients with ACHD and elevated PVR, there are several important management considerations in the setting of HF. Some of these considerations are relevant to specific congenital anatomies, whereas others represent more general principles that inform patient management.

Eisenmenger Syndrome

ES is encountered most often in the setting of large, unrepaired ASD or VSD, although it may also occur in the setting of more complex CHD that includes systemic-to-pulmonary shunts.[18] Once pulmonary vascular disease has progressed to the extent that pulmonary resistance is higher than systemic resistance, the shunt reverses and progressive hypoxemia leads to ES, a multisystemic condition variably associated with HF, arrhythmia, renal dysfunction, erythrocytosis, hyperviscosity, thrombocytopenia, coagulopathy, iron deficiency, gout, gallstones, and osteoarthropathy.[37–42] Discussion of the management of all aspects of ES is beyond the scope of this review. Given that HF presents in ES with a broad symptomatology, this discussion focuses specifically on the management of elevated PVR in the setting of symptomatic ES.

In ES, the systemic CO is preserved at the expense of worsening hypoxia from right-to-left shunting. Targeted PAH therapies have been investigated in the management of symptomatic ES, and randomized clinical trials (RCTs) have established the safety and efficacy of several different drug classes. Agent selection and timing, dose titration, and indications for altering strategy have not yet been fully established. Given the absence of these data, recommendations from current society guidelines are primarily based on expert opinion.[7,33,43]

The endothelin receptor antagonist (ERA), bosentan, was the first targeted PAH therapy studied in ES. In BREATH-5, the initial RCT in ES, a decrease in mPAP and indexed PVR were seen, as well as improved 6-minute walk distance (6MWD) with bosentan, without any decrease in Sao_2.[44] Subsequent trials have supported these beneficial effects, along with sustained long-term improvement, supporting its first-line use in symptomatic ES.[33,45] In the 2019 RCT, MAESTRO, macitentan did not improve 6MWD after 16 weeks of therapy, although the hemodynamic substudy did show a reduction in indexed PVR.[46] Several small RCTs and prospective trials have shown decreases in PVR, improved effective Qp, and improved functional class with phosphodiesterase type 5 (PDE-5) inhibitors.[47,48] Last, there are some data supporting the safety and efficacy of inhaled prostanoids in symptomatic ES.[49]

Similar to other forms of ACHD-HF, identifying the onset of symptoms is challenging in ES. Although many patients with ES deny symptoms, significant exercise limitations are universally seen during cardiopulmonary exercise testing, and many experts think that early initiation of PAH therapies in these patients is likely to provide the most benefit.[50] For those with significant activity limitations, combination therapy with the addition of PDE-5 inhibitors or prostanoids may be of greater benefit.[51–54] Despite conflicting evidence for up-front prostanoid-containing combination therapy, in a trial of 28 patients with ES experiencing suboptimal disease control on dual-agent oral therapy with an ERA and a PDE-5 inhibitor, addition of a parenteral prostanoid (subcutaneous treprostinil or intravenous epoprostenol) resulted in improved functional class, 6MWD, and decreased N-terminal probrain natriuretic peptide (NT-proBNP) levels.[55] As a specific form of ACHD-HF with elevated PVR, ES requires management by a multidisciplinary care team led by CHD physicians, with a focus on the early identification of decompensation and implementation of targeted treatment approaches.

Fontan Circulation

For patients born with single-ventricle anatomy, the Fontan correction has facilitated survival well into adulthood. Elevated PVR is one of the established mechanisms of Fontan failure; in a circulation devoid of a subpulmonic pump, any increase in PVR is generally poorly tolerated. It has been proposed that the pulmonary arterial vascular bed represents the "critical bottleneck" of the Fontan circulation, characterized by obligatory upstream congestion and downstream reduced flows.[56] Although ventricular failure does occur in the Fontan circulation, this is thought to represent a minority of cases, with most cases of circulatory failure related to factors independent of the single ventricle's function. Elevated PVR is one important driver of Fontan failure. Models suggest that significant pulmonary vessel derecruitment occurs in the setting of nonpulsatile pulmonary flow that is present in the Fontan circulation. These effects lead to a systematic underappreciation of true PVR by as much as 30% according to conventional measurement techniques.[57] Despite the role of elevated PVR in Fontan failure, data supporting the use of pulmonary vasodilators for the management of Fontan failure remains limited.[58] Although studies to date demonstrate good tolerance of ERAs and PDE-5 inhibitors, with some improvements in exercise parameters, hemodynamics, and symptoms, only one randomized trial has shown a significant improvement in its primary endpoint, and no studies to date have demonstrated sustained improvements in NT-proBNP levels, quality of life, or reductions in morbidity/mortality.[58] Interestingly, most studies have not specifically targeted patients with elevated PVR. The currently enrolling Single Ventricle Interventional Trial is assessing the benefit of sildenafil in patients with mean PAP greater than 15 mm Hg and transpulmonary gradient greater than 5 mm Hg and may revive interest in this drug class if successful.[59]

Mixed Group 2 Disease

In contrast to specific CHD structural and functional considerations above, a more general consideration of the management of ACHD-HF in the setting of elevated PVR is the consideration of mixed Group 2 disease. This describes instances in which PCWP is high, but the PVR is elevated disproportionately. This may occur in the setting of incipient HF in those with preexisting precapillary PH or in those with longstanding pulmonary congestion in which a "reactive" phase of their Group 2 PH is thought to induce precapillary remodeling.[19]

Recognition of these overlapping PH causes is particularly important given evidence trending toward harm if these patients receive targeted PAH therapies, particularly ERAs.[60–63] These harms are thought to be related to precipitation of pulmonary edema and volume overload related to an improved intrapulmonary circulation overloading the failing systemic ventricle. Two of the initial trials investigating ERAs in Group 2 disease were terminated early or the study drug was discontinued early because of trends toward increased adverse events in the treatment arms.[60,63] Although there is some exciting evidence regarding possible benefits of the use of PDE-5 inhibitors and soluble guanylate cyclase stimulators in Group 2 PH, none of these studies have enrolled patients with ACHD-HF.[61 69] Given these findings, management of mixed Group 2 PH in the setting of ACHD-HF focuses on excellent management of patients' HF, characterized by normalization of systemic ventricular filling pressures, followed by consideration of defect closure and/or targeted PAH therapies.

Defect Closure

For patients with ACHD-PAH and intracardiac or extracardiac shunts that have not progressed to ES, defect closure may halt the progression of PAH and allow for disease reversal in carefully selected cases. Although several studies have demonstrated a decrease in PAH prevalence as well as reduction in pulmonary arterial pressures following ASD closure, shunt closure is not appropriate for all patients and must be carefully considered.[70] For instance, in patients that have progressed to early ES, their defect can facilitate both pressure and volume offloading of the subpulmonary ventricle in the setting of significantly elevated PVRs. Defect closure in these cases could exacerbate right HF, leading to total cardiovascular collapse and death. Given this, as defect closure is considered, patients should be closely monitored for exercise-induced desaturation. Inducible right-to-left shunting indicates that with small elevations in PVR, the defects are serving a pressure and volume offloading function for the subpulmonary ventricle, and defect closure should not be recommended. Notably, for patients with patent ductus arteriosus or other shunts distal to the upper extremity blood supply, exercise-induced desaturation should be assessed for by measurements in the lower extremities. For patients with small or coincidental shunts, defect closure is not recommended given that closure is unlikely to affect the natural history of their PAH, and because the closure procedure is not without potential complications.

This leaves as candidates for defect closure a subset of patients with moderate to large unrepaired defects with evidence of PAH who have not yet progressed to ES. Guidelines currently recommend defect closure as a Class I recommendation only for symptomatic patients with PVR less than one-third of systemic vascular resistance, PA systolic pressure less the half of systemic systolic pressure, and Qp:Qs greater than or equal to 1.5:1.[33]

Targeted Pulmonary Arterial Hypertension Therapies

For those with ACHD-HF in the setting of elevated PVR, following the appropriate management of Group 2 PH contributions, targeted therapies for residual PAH may be considered. For pre-tricuspid lesions, the addition of PAH therapies is often well tolerated. For those with post-tricuspid lesions, especially those who are actively being managed for HF, any future addition of PAH therapies must occur in a closely monitored setting out of caution for precipitating pressure or volume overload of the systemic ventricle and subsequent pulmonary edema and/or worsening of left-to-right shunting.

As noted for the management of ES, bosentan is the most studied ERA in ACHD, with multiple short- and long-term studies demonstrating safety, tolerability, hemodynamic benefits, and improvements in 6MWD.[71–77] Nearly all of these prior studies have excluded patients with reduced systemic ventricular function. In light of earlier data investigating ERAs in Group 2 disease that trended toward harm, the safety and efficacy of these agents for the management of elevated PVR in patients with ACHD-HF remain unknown.

PDE-5 inhibitors have also been studied in the management of elevated PVR in ACHD, with several trials demonstrating improved function status and 6MWD.[78,79] As previously noted, PDE-5 inhibitors as part of combination therapy in ES have demonstrated good tolerability and improved hemodynamics and function status.[47,48] Although not explicitly studied in HF, the evidence supporting safety of PDE-5 inhibitors in Group 2 PH may translate to managing elevated PVR in ACHD-HF.[64–68] Current guidelines recommend the use of PDE-5 inhibitors in patients with ACHD-PAH and insufficient symptomatic improvement with single-drug therapy.[33]

There is very limited data to guide the appropriate medical management of segmental PAH. It is important to note the possibility of worsening ventilation/perfusion (V/Q) matching and resultant hypoxemia with parenteral or oral treatments. This is related to the nonselective vasodilation of capillary bed receiving perfusion, irrespective of whether they receive adequate ventilation. Although this physiology can be encountered in any type of PAH, there are numerous case reports demonstrating this in segmental PAH.[80,81] Inhalational administration of advanced therapies delivers medication selectively to segments receiving adequate ventilation, decreasing the likelihood of worsening V/Q mismatch and potentially improving V/Q matching. To date, few inhaled therapies have been studied in ACHD-PAH, particularly in the context of HF.

Mechanical Circulatory Support

Uncertainty remains about the proper use and timing of both mechanical circulatory support (MCS) and transplantation in ACHD-HF, owing to a still emerging evidence base comprising largely case reports, case series, and retrospective registry studies. In the setting of HF, patients with ACHD are known to experience low use of MCS despite contemporary data demonstrating dramatically expanded use of MCS in HF among their non-ACHD peers.[82–84] Increasingly, MCS is being used as a bridge to transplantation with a recent report demonstrating nearly half of all adult patients with HF transplanted off of MCS.[85] This trend appears to be almost exclusively driven by non-ACHD-HF, given that patients with ACHD constitute less than 1% of all patients supported by durable MCS, per data from the INTERMACS (Interagency Registry for Mechanically Assisted Circulatory Support).[82]

This lower utilization of MCS in patients with ACHD may be expected given that most forms of MCS were developed to support typical cardiac anatomy and are often not transposable to the many ACHD anatomies that may require support. Furthermore, knowledge gaps remain regarding the fundamental hemodynamics of many ACHD anatomies, particularly the palliated Fontan circulation, complicating the application of MCS to instances of circulatory failure. Given the paucity of data regarding the timing and use of MCS in ACHD-HF, even less is certain regarding the use of MCS in the setting of elevated PVR. Although a comprehensive discussion of MCS selection is beyond the scope of this review, clinicians should ideally consider 3 factors when evaluating the role of MCS in the setting of ACHD-HF. The first of these is clear articulation of which structure or structures require support (univentricular support of the systemic ventricle or subpulmonary ventricle, biventricular support, univentricular support of a single ventricular circulation mindful of its morphologic origin). Second, the duration of support should be considered before MCS initiation (short term or long term; <14 days is often referred to as short term). Third, the need for membrane oxygenation should be evaluated. Together these

3 considerations can substantially clarify device selection and clinical strategy.

Transplantation

Transplantation remains an important consideration for patients with ACHD experiencing advanced HF. Although a full review of transplantation in the setting of ACHD-HF is beyond the scope of this review, several disparities deserve highlighting. According to United Network for Organ Sharing data, patients with ACHD listed for transplant are less likely than their non-ACHD peers to receive a transplant (53% vs 64%).[86] In addition to having longer wait times, these data demonstrate that patients with ACHD were less likely to receive a transplant at every time interval after listing and for each priority tier compared with their non-ACHD peers.[86]

Patients with ACHD encounter many challenges that drive disparate organ allocation and wait times. Several of these are structurally engrained within listing priority assessments based on assumptions about disease severity founded in non-ACHD-HF pathophysiology and therapies; as above, MCS utilization is less common in ACHD-HF, which significantly disadvantages the listing priority of these patients. Other device therapies that have demonstrated improved outcomes in non-ACHD-HF; for instance, implantable cardiac defibrillators (ICD) and cardiac resynchronization therapy, have not been fully validated in patients with ACHD, resulting in significantly lower utilization, with one large registry demonstrating the presence of ICDs in 75% in non-ACHD patients compared with 44% in patients with ACHD by the time of transplant.[3] In addition, ejection fraction (EF)-based cutoffs, established from the study of non-ACHD-HF populations, often have poor application to ACHD-HF, where ventricular EF may be normal or near normal despite advanced HF, impacting device candidacy and objective assessments of disease severity.

Other disease-specific elements influence listing wait times, primarily by limiting the donor pool, including the ACHD patient's greater predilection for allosensitization, given increased frequency of prior blood transfusions and implantation of graft materials related to prior palliative surgeries, as well as surgical-anatomical needs of patients with ACHD, which may require greater lengths of donor tissue and vessels for intraoperative reconstruction.[87,88]

Following successful listing and organ transplantation, patients with ACHD experience higher 1-year mortality than their non-ACHD peers, although subsequently enjoy superior long-term survival.[85,89] According to data from the International Society for Heart and Lung Transplantation, between the years of 1985 and 2010, ACHD transplant survival at 1, 5, 10, and 15 years was 77%, 67%, 57%, and 53%, respectively, compared with their non-ACHD peers' survival at these intervals of 83%, 70%, 53%, and 37%.[89] Reasons for high 1-year mortality in patients with ACHD are thought to be related to multiple factors, including longer ischemic times owing in part to prior sternotomies and need of additional intraoperative reconstruction, as well as higher incidence of primary graft failure, multiorgan failure, stroke, posttransplant renal failure requiring dialysis, and need for reoperation.[90,91] In addition, patient age is a predictor of 1-year mortality with a peak at 25 to 30 years[89,92]; these individuals are also known to have a lower death rate owing to infection, possibly implicating a more robust immune system, which may be more challenging to control with standard immunosuppression regimens.[92] This is only compounded by this age group's challenge with medication adherence.[93] These non-perioperative factors broaden the lens on needed health care interventions to address higher 1-year mortality for patients with ACHD receiving transplantation.

There remains no formal guidance that specifically addresses clear selection criteria for heart versus heart-lung transplantation in patients with ACHD. Furthermore, as discussed above, the assessment of PVR in these patients can be challenging even when they are healthy and is only made more challenging in the setting of HF. These limitations make it particularly challenging to predict beforehand the "unmasking" of elevated PVRs posttransplant as the new healthy subpulmonary ventricle mounts an improved cardiac output that is partially flow limited by the true PVR.[94,95] Several groups have reported success in overcoming this outcome by intentionally oversizing donor hearts.[88,96]

SUMMARY

The presence of elevated PVR dramatically increases the complexity of management in patients with ACHD-HF. Already a challenging condition to define, ACHD-HF often incorporates specific anatomies, including intracardiac and extracardiac shunts, that require rigorous diagnostic characterization and heighten the importance of considering overall hemodynamic impacts of modifying pulmonary and systemic vascular resistance. Total circulatory management in patients with ACHD-HF requires input from multidisciplinary care teams availing the use of medical, interventional, and surgical approaches. As the prevalence of ACHD steadily increases, future studies will be needed to advance the understanding of the management of elevated PVR in ACHD-HF.

CLINICS CARE POINTS

- Adults with Congenital Heart Disease (ACHD) can experience several different types of pulmonary hypertension (PH) comorbid with their known cardiac lesions. Given the vulnerability of ACHD hearts to developing heart failure (ACHD-HF), many patients will experience some degree of World Health Organization (WHO) Group 2 PH.

- Invasive hemodynamics (by right heart catheterization) may reveal elevated pulmonary vascular resistance (PVR) above what can be explained by elevated systemic ventricular filling pressures.

- The specific management of elevated PVR in the setting of ACHD-HF requires rigorous characterization of intracardiac, intrapulmonary, and other vascular anatomy along with invasive assessment of the hemodynamic significance of identified lesions. Transthoracic echocardiography, cardiac magnetic resonance imaging, and heart catheterization are important modalities used to assess structure, function, and hemodynamic effects.

- Therapies to address elevated PVR in the setting of ACHD-HF include pharmacologic, catheter-based interventions, and surgical strategies. These often center around reducing the contribution of existing group 2 disease prior to addressing the overlay of other of forms of PH.

- Total circulatory management in patients with ACHD-HF and elevated PVR requires input from multidisciplinary care teams availing the use of medical, interventional, and surgical approaches.

DISCLOSURE

Dr. Krasuski serves as a consultant for Actelion/Janssen Pharmaceuticals, Bayer, Neptune Medical and Gore Medical. He receives research funding from the Adult Congenital Heart Association and Actelion/Janssen Pharmaceuticals and serves as an investigator for Edwards Lifesciences and Medtronic. Dr. Kusner reports no conflicts.

REFERENCES

1. Warnes CA, Liberthson R, Danielson GK, et al. Task force 1: the changing profile of congenital heart disease in adult life. J Am Coll Cardiol 2001;37(5):1170–5.
2. Oliver JM, Gallego P, Gonzalez AE, et al. Risk factors for excess mortality in adults with congenital heart diseases. Eur Heart J 2017;38(16):1233–41.
3. Verheugt CL, Uiterwaal CSPM, Van Der Velde ET, et al. Mortality in adult congenital heart disease. Eur Heart J 2010;31(10):1220–9.
4. Lui GK, Fernandes S, McElhinney DB. Management of cardiovascular risk factors in adults with congenital heart disease. J Am Heart Assoc 2014;3(6):1–9.
5. Lowe BS, Therrien J, Ionescu-Ittu R, et al. Diagnosis of pulmonary hypertension in the congenital heart disease adult population: Impact on outcomes. J Am Coll Cardiol 2011;58(5):538–46.
6. Simonneau G, Montani D, Celermajer DS, et al. Haemodynamic definitions and updated clinical classification of pulmonary hypertension. Eur Respir J 2019;53(1).
7. Humbert M, Kovacs G, Hoeper MM, et al. 2022 ESC/ERS Guidelines for the Diagnosis and Treatment of Pulmonary Hypertension Developed by the Task Force for the Diagnosis and Treatment of (ESC) and the European Respiratory Society (ERS). Eur Heart J 2022;00:1–114.
8. Papamichalis M, Xanthopoulos A, Papamichalis P, et al. Adult congenital heart disease with pulmonary arterial hypertension: mechanisms and management. Heart Fail Rev 2020;25(5):773–94.
9. Harrison RE, Berger R, Haworth SG, et al. Transforming growth factor-β receptor mutations and pulmonary arterial hypertension in childhood. Circulation 2005;111(4):435–41.
10. Diller GP, Gatzoulis MA. Pulmonary vascular disease in adults with congenital heart disease. Circulation 2007;115(8):1039–50.
11. HEATH D, EDWARDS JE. The pathology of hypertensive pulmonary vascular disease; a description of six grades of structural changes in the pulmonary arteries with special reference to congenital cardiac septal defects. Circulation 1958;18(4 Part 1):533–47.
12. Rabinovitch M, Haworth SG, Castaneda AR, et al. Lung biopsy in congenital heart disease: A morphometric approach to pulmonary vascular disease. Circulation 1978;58(6):1107–22.
13. Haworth SG. Pulmonary hypertension in the young. Heart 2002;88(6):658–64.
14. Zamora MR, Stelzner TJ, Webb S, et al. Overexpression of endothelin-1 and enhanced growth of pulmonary artery smooth muscle cells from fawn-hooded rats. Am J Physiol Lung Cell Mol Physiol 1996;270(1 14–1).
15. Van Der Feen DE, Bartelds B, De Boer RA, et al. Assessment of reversibility in pulmonary arterial hypertension and congenital heart disease. Heart 2019;105(4):276–82.

16. Steele PM, Fuster V, Cohen M, et al. Isolated atrial septal defect with pulmonary vascular obstructive disease - long-term follow-up and prediction of outcome after surgical correction. Circulation 1987; 76(5):1037–42.

17. Kozlik-Feldmann R, Hansmann G, Bonnet D, et al. Pulmonary hypertension in children with congenital heart disease (PAH-CHD, PPHVD-CHD). Expert consensus statement on the diagnosis and treatment of paediatric pulmonary hypertension. The European Paediatric Pulmonary Vascular Disease Network, endorsed by ISHLT and DGPK. Heart 2016;102:II42–8.

18. Kempny A, Hjortshøj CS, Gu H, et al. Predictors of Death in Contemporary Adult Patients with Eisenmenger Syndrome: A Multicenter Study. Circulation 2017;135(15):1432–40.

19. Guazzi M, Borlaug BA. Pulmonary hypertension due to left heart disease. Circulation 2012;126(8):975–90.

20. Singh N, Dorfmüller P, Shlobin OA, et al. Group 3 Pulmonary Hypertension: From Bench to Bedside. Circ Res 2022;130(9):1404–22.

21. Hoeper MM, Mayer E, Simonneau G, et al. Chronic thromboembolic pulmonary hypertension. Circulation 2006;113(16):2011–20.

22. Morgenstern I, Kauczor H. Bronchopulmonary Shunts in Thromboembolic Pulmonary Hypertension: Evaluation with Helical. 2002;(November): 1209-1215.

23. Endrys J, Hayat N, Cherian G. Comparison of bronchopulmonary collaterals and collateral blood flow in patients with chronic thromboembolic and primary pulmonary hypertension. Heart 1997;78(2):171–6.

24. Johnson RJ, Haworth SG. Pulmonary vascular and alveolar development in tetralogy of Fallot: A recommendation for early correction. Thorax 1982;37(12): 893–901.

25. Haworth SG, Reid L. Quantitative structural study of pulmonary circulation in the newborn with pulmonary atresia. Thorax 1977;32(2):129–33.

26. van Albada ME, Schoemaker RG, Kemna MS, et al. The role of increased pulmonary blood flow in pulmonary arterial hypertension. Eur Respir J 2005; 26(3):487–93.

27. Wood P. The Eisenmenger Syndrome or Pulmonary Hypertension with Reversed Central Shunt. Br Med J 1958;2(5099):755.

28. Young D, Mark H. Fate of the patient with the Eisenmenger syndrome. Am J Cardiol 1971;28(6):658–69.

29. Duffels MGJ, Engelfriet PM, Berger RMF, et al. Pulmonary arterial hypertension in congenital heart disease: An epidemiologic perspective from a Dutch registry. Int J Cardiol 2007;120(2):198–204.

30. Simonneau G, Gatzoulis MA, Adatia I, et al. Updated clinical classification of pulmonary hypertension. J Am Coll Cardiol 2013;62(25 SUPPL).

31. Lammers AE, Bauer LJ, Diller GP, et al. Pulmonary hypertension after shunt closure in patients with simple congenital heart defects. Int J Cardiol 2020; 308:28–32.

32. Çelik M, Yılmaz Y, Küp A, et al. Predictors of pulmonary hypertension after atrial septal defect closure: Impact of atrial fibrillation. Turkish J Thorac Cardiovasc Surg 2022;30(3):344–53.

33. Stout KK, Daniels CJ, Aboulhosn JA, et al. 2018 AHA/ACC Guideline for the Management of Adults With Congenital Heart Disease: A Report of the American College of Cardiology/American Heart Association Task Force on Clinical Practice Guidelines. Vol 139.; 2019. doi:10.1161/CIR.0000000000000603.

34. Manes A, Palazzini M, Leci E, et al. Current era survival of patients with pulmonary arterial hypertension associated with congenital heart disease: A comparison between clinical subgroups. Eur Heart J 2014;35(11):716–24.

35. Rudski LG, Lai WW, Afilalo J, et al. Guidelines for the Echocardiographic Assessment of the Right Heart in Adults: A Report from the American Society of Echocardiography. Endorsed by the European Association of Echocardiography, a registered branch of the European Society of Cardiology, and the Canadian Society of Echocardiography. J Am Soc Echocardiogr 2010;23(7):685–713.

36. Landzberg MJ, Daniels CJ, Forfia P, et al. Timely PAH Identification in Adults With Repaired Congenital Heart Disease? The ACHD-QuERI Registry Insights. JACC Adv 2023;2(9):100649.

37. Baskar S, Horne P, Fitzsimmons S, et al. Arrhythmia burden and related outcomes in Eisenmenger syndrome. Congenit Heart Dis 2017;12(4):512–9.

38. Westbury SK, Lee K, Reilly-Stitt C, et al. High haematocrit in cyanotic congenital heart disease affects how fibrinogen activity is determined by rotational thromboelastometry. Thromb Res 2013;132(2):e145–51.

39. Jensen AS, Johansson PI, Bochsen L, et al. Fibrinogen function is impaired in whole blood from patients with cyanotic congenital heart disease. Int J Cardiol 2013;167(5):2210–4.

40. Diller GP, Dimopoulos K, Broberg CS, et al. Presentation, survival prospects, and predictors of death in Eisenmenger syndrome: A combined retrospective and case-control study. Eur Heart J 2006;27(14):1737–42.

41. Dimopoulos K, Diller GP, Koltsida E, et al. Prevalence, predictors, and prognostic value of renal dysfunction in adults with congenital heart disease. Circulation 2008;117(18):2320–8.

42. Oya H, Nagaya N, Satoh T, et al. Haemodynamic correlates and prognostic significance of serum uric acid in adult patients with Eisenmenger syndrome. Heart 2000;84(1):53–8.

43. Baumgartner H, de Backer J, Babu-Narayan SV, et al. 2020 ESC Guidelines for the management of adult congenital heart disease. Eur Heart J 2021;42(6): 563–645.

44. Galiè N, Beghetti M, Gatzoulis MA, et al. Bosentan therapy in patients with Eisenmenger syndrome: A

multicenter, double-blind, randomized, placebo-controlled study. Circulation 2006;114(1):48–54.

45. Baumgartner H, Falk V, Bax JJ, et al. 2017 ESC/EACTS Guidelines for the management of valvular heart disease. Eur Heart J 2017;38(36):2739–91.

46. Gatzoulis MA, Landzberg M, Beghetti M, et al. Evaluation of Macitentan in Patients with Eisenmenger Syndrome: Results from the Randomized, Controlled MAESTRO Study. Circulation 2019;139(1):51–63.

47. Mukhopadhyay S, Nathani S, Yusuf J, et al. Clinical efficacy of phosphodiesterase-5 inhibitor tadalafil in Eisenmenger Syndrome—A randomized, placebo-controlled, double-blind crossover study. Congenit Heart Dis 2011;6(5):424–31.

48. Singh TP, Rohit M, Grover A, et al. A randomized, placebo-controlled, double-blind, crossover study to evaluate the efficacy of oral sildenafil therapy in severe pulmonary artery hypertension. Am Heart J 2006;151(4):851.e1–5.

49. Nashat H, Kempny A, Harries C, et al. A single-centre, placebo-controlled, double-blind randomised cross-over study of nebulised iloprost in patients with Eisenmenger syndrome: A pilot study. Int J Cardiol 2020;299:131–5.

50. Kempny A, Dimopoulos K, Uebing A, et al. Reference values for exercise limitations among adults with congenital heart disease. Relation to activities of daily lifesingle centre experience and review of published data. Eur Heart J 2012;33(11):1386–96.

51. Iversen K, Jensen AS, Jensen TV, et al. Combination therapy with bosentan and sildenafil in Eisenmenger syndrome: A randomized, placebo-controlled, double-blinded trial. Eur Heart J 2010;31(9):1124–31.

52. Hoeper MM, Leuchte H, Halank M, et al. Combining inhaled iloprost with bosentan in patients with idiopathic pulmonary arterial hypertension. Eur Respir J 2006;28(4):691–4.

53. Humbert M, Barst RJ, Robbins IM, et al. Combination of bosentan with epoprostenol in pulmonary arterial hypertension: BREATHE-2. Eur Respir J 2004;24(3):353–9.

54. McLaughlin VV, Oudiz RJ, Frost A, et al. Randomized study of adding inhaled iloprost to existing bosentan in pulmonary arterial hypertension. Am J Respir Crit Care Med 2006;174(11):1257–63.

55. D'Alto M, Constantine A, Balint OH, et al. The effects of parenteral prostacyclin therapy as add-on treatment to oral compounds in Eisenmenger syndrome. Eur Respir J 2019;54(5):2–5.

56. Gewillig M, Brown SC. The Fontan circulation after 45 years: Update in physiology. Heart 2016;102(14):1081–6.

57. Jolley M, Colan SD, Rhodes J, et al. Fontan physiology revisited. Anesth Analg 2015;121(1):172–82.

58. Wang W, Hu X, Liao W, et al. The efficacy and safety of pulmonary vasodilators in patients with Fontan circulation: a meta-analysis of randomized controlled trials. Pulm Circ 2019;9(1).

59. Amedro P, Gavotto A, Abassi H, et al. Efficacy of phosphodiesterase type 5 inhibitors in univentricular congenital heart disease: the SV-INHIBITION study design. ESC Hear Fail 2020;7(2):747–56.

60. Califf RM, Adams KF, McKenna WJ, et al. A randomized controlled trial of epoprostenol therapy for severe congestive heart failure: The Flolan International Randomized Survival Trial (FIRST). Am Heart J 1997;134(1):44–54.

61. Lüscher TF, Enseleit F, Pacher R, et al. Hemodynamic and neurohumoral effects of selective endothelin A (ETA) receptor blockade in chronic heart failure: The heart failure ETA receptor blockade trial (HEAT). Circulation 2002;106(21):2666–72.

62. Anand PI, McMurray PJ, Cohn PJN, et al. Long-term effects of darusentan on left-ventricular remodelling and clinical outcomes in the EndothelinA Receptor Antagonist Trial in Heart Failure (EARTH): Randomised, double-blind, placebo-controlled trial. Lancet 2004;364(9431):347–54.

63. Kaluski E, Cotter G, Leitman M, et al. Clinical and hemodynamic effects of bosentan dose optimization in symptomatic heart failure patients with severe systolic dysfunction, associated with secondary pulmonary hypertension—A multi-center randomized study. Cardiology 2008;109(4):273–80.

64. Guazzi M, Vicenzi M, Arena R, et al. Pulmonary hypertension in heart failure with preserved ejection fraction: A target of phosphodiesterase-5 inhibition in a 1-year study. Circulation 2011;124(2):164–74.

65. Redfield MM, Chen HH, Borlaug BA, et al. Effect of phosphodiesterase-5 inhibition on exercise capacity and clinical status in heart failure with preserved ejection fraction: A randomized clinical trial. JAMA 2013;309(12):1268–77.

66. Hoendermis ES, Liu LCY, Hummel YM, et al. Effects of sildenafil on invasive haemodynamics and exercise capacity in heart failure patients with preserved ejection fraction and pulmonary hypertension: A randomized controlled trial. Eur Heart J 2015;36(38):2565–73.

67. Lewis GD, Shah R, Shahzad K, et al. Sildenafil improves exercise capacity and quality of life in patients with systolic heart failure and secondary pulmonary hypertension. Circulation 2007;116(14):1555–62.

68. Behling A, Rohde LE, Colombo FC, et al. Effects of 5′-Phosphodiesterase Four-Week Long Inhibition With Sildenafil in Patients With Chronic Heart Failure: A Double-Blind, Placebo-Controlled Clinical Trial. J Card Fail 2008;14(3):189–97.

69. Bonderman D, Ghio S, Felix SB, et al. Riociguat for patients with pulmonary hypertension caused by systolic left ventricular dysfunction: A phase IIb double-blind, randomized, placebo-controlled, dose-ranging hemodynamic study. Circulation 2013;128(5):502–11.

70. Zwijnenburg RD, Baggen VJM, Geenen LW, et al. The prevalence of pulmonary arterial hypertension before and after atrial septal defect closure at adult age: A systematic review. Am Heart J 2018;201: 63–71.

71. Ibrahim R, Granton JT, Mehta S. An open-label, multicentre pilot study of bosentan in pulmonary arterial hypertension related to congenital heart disease. Cancer Res J 2006;13(8):415–20.

72. Gatzoulis MA, Rogers P, Li W, et al. Safety and tolerability of bosentan in adults with Eisenmenger physiology. Int J Cardiol 2005;98(1):147–51.

73. Benza RL, Rayburn BK, Tallaj JA, et al. Efficacy of bosentan in a small cohort of adult patients with pulmonary arterial hypertension related to congenital heart disease. Chest 2006;129(4):1009–15.

74. Kotlyar E, Sy R, Keogh AM, et al. Bosentan for the treatment of pulmonary arterial hypertension associated with congenital cardiac disease. Cardiol Young 2006;16(3):268–74.

75. Schulze-Neick I, Gilbert N, Ewert R, et al. Adult patients with congenital heart disease and pulmonary arterial hypertension: First open prospective multicenter study of bosentan therapy. Am Heart J 2005;150(4). 716.e7.

76. D'Alto M, Vizza CD, Romeo E, et al. Long term effects of bosentan treatment in adult patients with pulmonary arterial hypertension related to congenital heart disease (Eisenmenger physiology): Safety, tolerability, clinical, and haemodynamic effect. Heart 2007;93(5):621–5.

77. Diller GP, Dimopoulos K, Kaya MG, et al. Long-term safety, tolerability and efficacy of bosentan in adults with pulmonary arterial hypertension associated with congenital heart disease. Heart 2007;93(8):974–6.

78. Mukhopadhyay S, Sharma M, Ramakrishnan S, et al. Phosphodiesterase-5 inhibitor in Eisenmenger syndrome: A preliminary observational study. Circulation 2006;114(17):1807–10.

79. Zeng WJ, Lu XL, Xiong CM, et al. The efficacy and safety of sildenafil in patients with pulmonary arterial hypertension associated with the different types of congenital heart disease. Clin Cardiol 2011;34(8): 513–8.

80. Yasuhara J, Yamagishi H. Pulmonary arterial hypertension associated with tetralogy of Fallot. Int Heart J 2015;56:S17–21.

81. Grant EK, Berger JT. Use of Pulmonary Hypertension Medications in Patients with Tetralogy of Fallot with Pulmonary Atresia and Multiple Aortopulmonary Collaterals. Pediatr Cardiol 2016;37(2):304–12.

82. Bowen RES, Graetz TJ, Emmert DA, et al. Statistics of heart failure and mechanical circulatory support in 2020. Ann Transl Med 2020;8(13):827.

83. Gelow JM, Song HK, Weiss JB, et al. Organ allocation in adults with congenital heart disease listed for heart transplant: Impact of ventricular assist devices. J Heart Lung Transplant 2013;32(11):1059–64.

84. Alshawabkeh LI, Hu N, Carter KD, et al. Wait-List Outcomes for Adults With Congenital Heart Disease Listed for Heart Transplantation in the U.S. J Am Coll Cardiol 2016;68(9):908–17.

85. Lund LH, Khush KK, Cherikh WS, et al. The Registry of the International Society for Heart and Lung Transplantation: Thirty-fourth Adult Heart Transplantation Report—2017; Focus Theme: Allograft ischemic time. J Heart Lung Transplant 2017; 36(10):1037–46.

86. Everitt MD, Donaldson AE, Stehlik J, et al. Would access to device therapies improve transplant outcomes for adults with congenital heart disease? Analysis of the United Network for Organ Sharing (UNOS). J Heart Lung Transplant 2011;30(4): 395–401.

87. Cedars A, Vanderpluym C, Koehl D, et al. An Interagency Registry for Mechanically Assisted Circulatory Support (INTERMACS) analysis of hospitalization, functional status, and mortality after mechanical circulatory support in adults with congenital heart disease. J Heart Lung Transplant 2018;37(5):619–30.

88. Irving C, Parry G, O'Sullivan J, et al. Cardiac transplantation in adults with congenital heart disease. Heart 2010;96(15):1217–22.

89. Burchill LJ, Edwards LB, Dipchand AI, et al. Impact of adult congenital heart disease on survival and mortality after heart transplantation. J Heart Lung Transplant 2014;33(11):1157–63.

90. Patel ND, Weiss ES, Allen JG, et al. Heart Transplantation for Adults With Congenital Heart Disease: Analysis of the United Network for Organ Sharing Database. Ann Thorac Surg 2009;88(3):814–22.

91. Davies RR, Russo MJ, Yang J, et al. Listing and transplanting adults with congenital heart disease. Circulation 2011;123(7):759–67.

92. George JF, Taylor DO, Blume ED, et al. Minimizing infection and rejection death: Clues acquired from 19 years of multi institutional cardiac transplantation data. J Heart Lung Transplant 2011;30(2):151–7.

93. Foster BJ, Dahhou M, Zhang X, et al. Association between age and graft failure rates in young kidney transplant recipients. Transplantation 2011;92(11): 1237–43.

94. Mitchell MB, Campbell DN, Ivy D, et al. Evidence of pulmonary vascular disease after heart transplantation for Fontan circulation failure. J Thorac Cardiovasc Surg 2004;128(5):693–702.

95. Egbe AC, Connolly HM, Miranda WR, et al. Hemodynamics of Fontan Failure: The Role of Pulmonary Vascular Disease. Circ Hear Fail 2017;10(12):1–8.

96. Kenny LA, DeRita F, Nassar M, et al. Transplantation in the single ventricle population. Ann Cardiothorac Surg 2018;7(1):152–9.

Failing with Cyanosis-Heart Failure in End-Stage Unrepaired or Partially Palliated Congenital Heart Disease

Nael Aldweib, MD[a],*, Craig Broberg, MD, MS[a]

KEYWORDS

- Cyanosis • Heart failure • Systemic oxygen transport • Effective pulmonary blood flow

KEY POINTS

- Cyanotic congenital heart disease (CHD) can be categorized into 2 groups based on the location of pulmonary blood flow restriction, whether there is pulmonary stenosis or no stenosis.
- Heart failure in cyanotic CHD could be defined by evidence of inadequate tissue oxygen delivery.
- The goal of managing cyanotic CHD is to maximize oxygen delivery to the tissues, specifically hemoglobin, oxygen saturation, and cardiac output.

INTRODUCTION

For adults with unaddressed or partially treated cyanotic congenital heart disease (CHD), achieving biventricular or single ventricle repair is often not an option. Thus, cyanosis continues to be a way of life for them. As a result, the primary focus of treatment should center on enhancing oxygen delivery capabilities and minimizing myocardial injury. It is a systemic condition resulting from insufficient oxygen supply, damaging vital organs. This damage may manifest as issues such as coagulopathy, brain abscess, cerebral microemboli, hemoptysis, gout, renal dysfunction, and myocardial injury and dysfunction. Inevitably, most individuals surviving with cyanotic CHD will develop features of heart failure. Yet failure manifestations are different in cyanosis; thus, management strategies are significantly nuanced. This article explores the necessary adaptations to chronic cyanosis and elements that can lead to deterioration. Considerations into managing acute decompensated heart failure (ADHF) and chronic heart failure are explored. Furthermore, the article delves into advanced treatment alternatives and considerations for end-of-life care.

CYANOTIC CONGENITAL HEART DISEASE OVERVIEW
Prevalence

In general, the occurrence rate of major CHD stands at 1%.[1–3] The variety of interventional options available now means that cyanotic conditions are usually repaired or palliated such that cyanosis is avoided. Nevertheless, a subset of individuals with severe CHD remain untreated or only partially palliated and are still cyanotic.[4,5] Thus, they are among the rarest yet most complex of all congenital heart patients. Although overall prevalence is unknown, they probably comprise 5% to 10% of any adult congenital heart disease (ACHD) clinic population. In the Dutch registry involving patients across the ACHD spectrum, 1% was identified as cyanotic.[6] Yet, due to both

[a] Knight Cardiovascular Institute, Oregon Health and Science University, UHN-623181 Southwest Sam Jackson Park Road, Portland, OR 97239, USA

* Corresponding author. Knight Cardiovascular Institute, Oregon Health and Science University, UHN-623181 Southwest, Sam Jackson Park Road, Portland, OR 97239.

E-mail address: aldweib@ohsu.edu

Heart Failure Clin 20 (2024) 223–236
https://doi.org/10.1016/j.hfc.2023.12.008
1551-7136/24/© 2023 Elsevier Inc. All rights reserved.

broadening treatment options during the last several decades and the gradual attrition of patients with cyanosis, their numbers are gradually in decline.

Etiology: Anatomic and Physiologic Factors

Although most heart defects are categorized by their anatomy, cyanosis is a physiologic condition that may be present in any number of defects. In each case, however, there must be a communication that allows for the right-to-left shunting wherein deoxygenated/venous blood is shunted to the systemic circulation and conditions that favor flow to the systemic circulation at the expense of the pulmonary circulation.

Cyanotic CHD can be categorized into 2 groups based on the location of pulmonary blood flow (PBF) restriction, namely whether there is pulmonary stenosis, that is, restriction in the great arteries, or no stenosis, that is, restriction in the pulmonary arterioles or capillaries (Eisenmenger syndrome [ES]). A systolic ejection murmur during a physical examination can often identify the former, whereas the lack of a murmur usually denotes the latter. Differentiation is important because management decisions are often very different between these groups.

The first group, which could be present in almost any defect involving a right-to-left shunt, classically is encountered in patients with abnormal or underdeveloped pulmonary arteries such as severe uncorrected pulmonary stenosis (PS) (or pulmonary artery [PA] band) with a shunt (ie, not isolated PS), conotruncal abnormalities such as tetralogy of Fallot, pulmonary atresia with ventricular septal defect (VSD), or truncus arteriosus, perhaps with partial palliation procedures such as surgical shunts placed in the past. Uncorrected single ventricle patients may also fall into this category because some degree of pulmonary stenosis is common.

The second group often involves patients with more simple shunts in the setting of pulmonary hypertension. ES is defined as (1) the presence of an intracardiac or great artery communication, (2) elevated pulmonary vascular resistance (PVR), and (3) bidirectional shunting. Shunts could be interatrial septal defect (ASD), VSD, patent ductus arteriosus (PDA), atrioventricular septal defect (AVSD), or aortopulmonary window (AP window), among others.

Exception to the general rule about the presence or absence of a murmur can be found. A patient with an atrial level shunt and severe right ventricular dysfunction or tricuspid valve regurgitation (such as Ebstein anomaly) may be cyanotic without pulmonary hypertension or a loud outflow murmur. A patient with a persistent left superior vena cava (SVC) to the left atrium may be similar.

PATHOPHYSIOLOGY OF CYANOSIS: DISTINGUISHING FEATURES IN COMPARISON TO OTHER HEART FAILURE CONDITIONS
Defining "Heart Failure" in Cyanotic Heart Disease

Heart failure in adults with cyanotic CHD does not neatly fit the standard definition applied to adults with acquired heart failure.[7] This is primarily because the heart failure symptoms in these adults result from a combination of anatomic and physiologic factors, including hypoxemia and a reduced capacity to deliver oxygen to the body's tissues, and thus be completely unrelated to significant impairment in ventricular systolic or diastolic function as is typically understood to be the case when the term "heart failure" is applied.

However, heart failure is a clinical diagnosis, not one based on ventricular function, and patients with cyanosis frequently exhibit the clinical features suggestive of the designation. Although it is likely that myocardial injury and dysfunction both play a role in cyanotic CHD, the fundamental issue is the diminished delivery of oxygen to the tissues. This is evident through symptoms such as fatigue, lassitude, dyspnea, headaches, myalgias, and a cold sensation. Heart failure in cyanotic CHD, therefore, could be defined by evidence of inadequate tissue oxygen delivery. As such, components of oxygen delivery are worth exploring herein.

- Components of oxygen delivery (**Fig. 1**)

Oxygen is carried in the blood through 2 primary mechanisms: it can either be dissolved in the plasma, denoted by the O_2 partial pressure in millimeters of mercury (mm Hg), a relatively small quantity, or bound to hemoglobin, measured as percent oxygen saturation (SaO_2). The combined effect of these 2 mechanisms determines the overall oxygen content in the blood. The oxygen-carrying *capacity* of hemoglobin is 1.36 mL O_2/g. The *oxygen content* of the blood (mL O_2/mL blood) is its carrying capacity multiplied by the percent oxygen saturation (plus the quantity of dissolved oxygen, which is usually trivial). Thus, it can be calculated as follows:

(1.36 × percent saturation × Hemoglobin) + (Partial pressure of oxygen [Po_2] × 0.003)

This relationship demonstrates that in low oxygen saturation, oxygen content can be normalized by additional hemoglobin.

Systemic oxygen transport (SOT), called delivery of oxygen, is the total amount of oxygen delivered

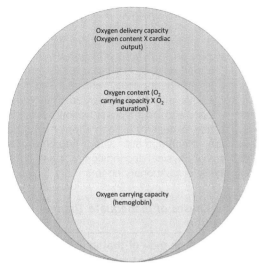

Fig. 1. Component of oxygen delivery to tissues.

to the systemic circulation. It is calculated by multiplying cardiac output by arterial oxygen content, expressed as cardiac output (mL blood/min) × oxygen content (mL O_2/mL blood), thus given in units of mL O_2/min. Ultimately, SOT must be maintained at an adequate level to ensure normal physiologic oxygen demands of the body (referred to as oxygen consumption [Vo_2]). Normal Oxygen delivery values may be 400 to 600 mL/min/m^2, with oxygen delivery 3 to 4 times Vo_2.[8] It is therefore an important therapeutic consideration in patients with cyanosis with signs of heart failure. This means that conditions wherein cardiac output is hindered will have a disadvantageous effect on SOT.

Although the term "cyanosis" used in this context is somewhat broadly applied, it technically refers only to skin color influenced by blood hue. The hemoglobin pigment changes its absorption of light based on whether it is oxygenated or deoxygenated, thus determining the color of the blood. Darker red is seen in typical venous blood with deoxyhemoglobin compared with arterial blood with oxyhemoglobin. A desaturation of at least 5 g/dL of hemoglobin must clinically manifest as cyanosis, specifically a bluish skin discoloration and mucous membranes.[9,10] Clinical definitions of "cyanosis" vary but usually indicate a resting arterial O_2 saturation of less than 90% at rest or less than 87% during activity. In contrast, hypoxia refers to low oxygen tension in the tissue, and hypoxemia refers to low oxygen content in arterial blood.

Some additional terms are worth defining here. PBF (Qp) denotes the total amount of blood traveling through the pulmonary capillary bed, and systemic blood flow (Qs, often called cardiac output)

denotes the amount reaching the systemic capillary bed. Effective blood flow (Qef) refers to the amount of deoxygenated blood that travels from the systemic capillary bed to the pulmonary capillary bed and vice versa, that is, without being shunted. Patients with cyanosis can remain stable despite variations in total PBF as long as their Qef remains above the individualized threshold for each patient. This amount is vital to maintain proper end-organ function and thus should be considered foremost in a failing patient with cyanosis.

Formulas to calculate flow states are shown in **Table 1**.

Normal Physiologic Adaptations to Cyanosis

Patients with cyanotic CHD have found a delicate balance that allows them to continue functioning despite the low oxygen content in their blood. Disruption of this homeostasis can have drastic consequences. To address inadequacies of tissue oxygen delivery in a struggling patient with cyanosis, it is necessary to understand the expected standard adaptations.

- *Erythropoiesis*

  Secondary erythrocytosis is the most important compensation for cyanosis. As the relationships discussed above demonstrate, elevated hemoglobin maintains oxygen content and, thus, SOT. Erythrocytosis is induced by hypoxia, which directly influences the bone marrow. Hypoxia triggers the expression of erythropoietin receptors, fostering erythropoiesis by regulating the maturation and proliferation of erythroid progenitors.[11,12] The hemoglobin concentration should be indirectly proportionate to the usual resting saturation and even indicate cyanosis severity for this exact reason.[10] Hemoglobin elevation is a vital response to cyanosis and should be left alone when present. Hemoglobin and hematocrit are important determinants of exercise capacity in cyanotic CHD.[13] Note that secondary erythrocytosis should not be misnamed "polycythemia," a term that implies propagation of leukocytes and platelets, usually not applicable in cyanotic CHD.

- *Arteriolar vasodilation and recruitment*

  Another important adaptation is the recruitment of arterioles. Hypoxemia and reduced blood oxygen content play a significant role in regulating blood vessel tone and structure. They have also been demonstrated to serve as powerful triggers for angiogenesis, a process in which new blood vessels develop from preexisting ones.[14] Hypoxia favors

Table 1
Formulas to calculate flow states and cardiac output

Qp or PBF	V_{O_2}/(Pulmonary Venous-Pulmonary Arterial Oxygen saturation) × oxygen Carrying Capacity
Qs or cardiac output	V_{O_2}/(pulmonary arterial-mixed venous oxygen saturation) × oxygen carrying capacity
Qef or effective PBF	V_{O_2}/(pulmonary venous-mixed venous oxygen saturation) × oxygen carrying capacity

V_{O_2} or oxygen consumption depends on metabolic state and can be either measured or estimated using various nomograms available

additional capillary recruitment locally through vascular endothelial growth factor (VEGF). VEGF encourages the proliferation of vascular endothelial cells in a paracrine fashion, forming new capillary vessels.[15] This can be seen, for example, as clubbing of the nail beds in cyanotics.

- *Increased oxygen utilization*

Oxygen becomes unbound to hemoglobin in environments with lower oxygen tension, such as tissue. This relationship, known as the oxyhemoglobin dissociation curve, is valuable for illustrating the relationship between these 2 crucial components. Various physiologic factors can alter the curve to favor dissociation earlier, that is, a right shift or raised p50 of the curve. This shift has been demonstrated in ES.[16] Cyanotic individuals have increased oxygen extraction at the tissue level, meaning they will have a lower venous oxygen saturation. This is especially true for the myocardium, which has the highest extraction per gram of tissue than any organ. It also makes it the most vulnerable to the effects of reduced oxygen delivery.

- *Hyperventilation*

Hyperventilation serves a crucial clinical role in response to low ambient oxygen, such as when living at high altitude. Gradually, however, respiration returns to normal as other compensations, such as erythrocytosis, become adequate. In cyanotic CHD, younger patients have been shown to have a respiratory alkalosis indicative of

hyperventilation, whereas this observation was less notable in older patients.[17] Although it is somewhat unclear what role chronic hyperventilation may play as an adaptation, altered ventilation should be avoided. CO_2 clearance is also affected by right-to-left shunts; thus, ventilation is vital. A failing cyanotic may be jeopardized by potential factors that lead to hypoventilation, such as narcotic use, excessive oxygen supplementation, restriction, diaphragmatic palsy, neuromuscular weakness or physical deconditioning, pneumonia, hemoptysis, or pulmonary edema.

Possible Causes of Inadequate Tissue Oxygenation

Given the importance of the adaptive measures described above, a compromise to any of them may affect the delicate balance of oxygen delivery to tissue and result in heart failure manifestations. Conditions that may precipitate an imbalance are worth considering (**Fig. 2**).

First is an imbalance of Qp and Qs, specifically an increase in PVR or decline in systemic vascular resistance (SVR), which will favor right-to-left shunting and worsen the cyanosis. Patients with cyanotic CHD who have limited PBF, either due to pulmonary arterial obstruction or increased PVR, may exhibit heart failure when tissue oxygenation becomes inadequate for physiologic needs. This might be due to worsening gradients through a pulmonary valve or insufficient collaterals, closure of a surgically created shunt, or even an increase in PVR. An imbalance can also be caused by anything that lowers SVR, such as sepsis, sedation medications, or massive allergic response for example. Whatever the cause, the imbalance worsens right-to-left shunting and hence oxygenation.

A second factor leading to deterioration is inadequate erythrocytosis. The process of secondary erythrocytosis is influenced by resting and exercise saturations, iron stores, vitamin B12, folic acid, erythropoietin levels, and the bone marrow condition. Erythrocytosis may be limited by any of these factors and jeopardize tissue oxygenation.

Third, chronic bleeding may lead to a suboptimal hemoglobin level. Common events include dental bleeding, epistaxis, and menorrhagia. Patients with cyanosis are also susceptible to recurrent hemoptysis, possibly from erosion of a dilated bronchial artery. It can be a cause of eventual death in 7% of the patients.[18] Chronic bleeding from any cause may be attributed to a combination of platelet disorders (including thrombocytopenia and thrombasthenia), abnormalities in coagulation pathways and impaired fibrinogen function.[19] Additionally, there may be reductions in vitamin

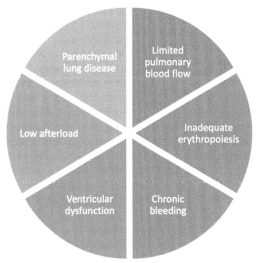

Fig. 2. Possible causes of inadequate tissue oxygenation.

K-dependent clotting factors and factor V, increased fibrinolytic activity, and depletion of the largest von Willebrand multimers.[20,21]

Fourth, ventricular dysfunction can worsen cardiac output and SOT or contribute to pulmonary edema and poor alveolar gas exchange. Because the myocardium has the highest oxygen extraction of any tissue, myocardial dysfunction gradually develops from chronic hypoxia. Ejection fraction and B-type natriuretic peptide are markers of poor prognosis.[22,23]

ACUTE DECOMPENSATED HEART FAILURE MANAGEMENT

Case Consideration: A 45-year-old man with Down syndrome, unrepaired complete atrioventricular canal defect with ES, has baseline saturations of 75% to 80%. He presented with viral pneumonia with saturations in the 50% range and altered mental status. BiPAP failed to improve his situation, acidosis worsened, and endotracheal intubation and mechanical ventilation were required. Treatment included antiviral agents and blood transfusions to maximize oxygen-carrying capacity and vasopressors to maintain SVR and minimize right-to-left shunting.

A critical message of this article is that the standard approach to left-sided heart failure in cyanotic individuals may not only be ineffective but also counterproductive and even dangerous. ADHF, from anything that disrupts the fragile homeostasis of a patient with cyanosis, may in and of itself be catastrophic and can increase the risk of mortality.[24] However, treatments such as intubation, diuresis, and afterload reduction, even

according to guideline-directed medical therapy, may all have significant drawbacks that can worsen the patient's already jeopardized condition. Because there is no reported experience in cyanosis with ADHF, any recommendation is based on an understanding of the above physiology and anecdotal experience. Potentially applicable strategies to consider are discussed here.

Identify Precipitating Factors

Reversing the inciting cause that triggers the ADHF event is crucial to reduce mortality. Once ADHF initiates, it sets off additional abnormalities affecting the heart, vasculature, neurohormonal system, kidneys, and liver in a cascade of organ dysfunction that may not be reversible. As such, isolating the initial trigger for deterioration can be difficult. Potential causes can be cardiovascular, such as arrhythmia, infective endocarditis, valvular heart disease, worsening PVR, or pulmonary arterial obstruction. However, they can also be extracardiac, such as respiratory illness, sepsis, hemoptysis or severe epistaxis, pulmonary thromboembolism, or new medications such as nonsteroidal anti-inflammatory drugs. Removal or resolution of the inciting event is the first step toward stabilization.

Maximize Systemic Oxygen Transport

The second goal in management is to maximize oxygen delivery to the tissues (**Fig. 3**). As discussed earlier, oxygen delivery, quantified as SOT, is the product of hemoglobin, oxygen saturation, and cardiac output. Therefore, these 3 factors offer important therapeutic targets and will be discussed individually.

- *Maintain hemoglobin*

Because secondary erythropoiesis is the mainstay of adaptation to cyanosis, an optimal hemoglobin level is paramount during acute decompensation. This is especially necessary to enhance oxygen delivery to the tissues when myocardial oxygen consumption is elevated and peripheral tissues have a heightened demand for oxygen. It is crucial to stimulate hemoglobin production through iron supplementation or transfusion to achieve this. Excessive hematocrit, however, can worsen viscosity.

The patient's historic levels should provide an optimal hemoglobin target during periods of stability and be indirectly correlated to their resting saturation.[16] In situations with an acute need to increase hemoglobin levels, blood transfusion can and should be considered, even though the measured hemoglobin is still within normal limits for the adult

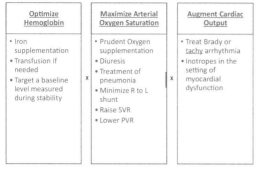

Fig. 3. Maximize systemic oxygen delivery to tissue.

population. There is no specific transfusion threshold or target; the approach should be tailored to each patient's unique needs. The primary objective of blood transfusion should be to see evidence of improved end-organ perfusion and clinical stability rather than achieve a certain number. Blood transfusion can be worthwhile for enhancing oxygen delivery when urgently needed.[25]

Therapeutic venesections should have no role in the management of deteriorating cyanotic CHD. They can lead to, or worsen, iron deficiency and decrease oxygen delivery to tissues, increasing the risk of cerebrovascular events and exacerbating heart failure.[26]

- *Maximize oxygen saturation*

Optimal saturation is addressed through 2 means: (1) improvement of alveolar gas exchange and (2) minimizing right-to-left shunt. The former means attention to pulmonary problems such as pneumonia or pulmonary edema, as well as the use of supplemental oxygen. The standard intensive care unit approach to deterioration and low arterial oxygen saturation often involves administering 100% oxygen to elevate partial oxygen pressure in the plasma. However, normalizing saturation is usually neither necessary nor achievable, and caution is needed to prevent suppression of the respiratory drive.

The later and often overlooked strategy should minimize right-to-left shunting to raise the arterial oxygen saturation levels. Shunts are driven by relative resistance in the pulmonary versus systemic circulation. Hence, sustaining a more favorable equilibrium between SVR and PVR is an important strategy for managing a decompensated patient with cyanosis. Importantly, this contrasts with the goals of afterload reduction in someone with myocardial dysfunction. A low SVR may be just as damaging as a high PVR and should be avoided.

The strategy is to paradoxically increase systemic arterial blood pressure by avoiding vasodilators and using vasopressors. When SVR is higher

than PVR, it should favor more left-to-right rather than right-to-left shunting and help restore balance to the jeopardized patient with cyanosis. One primary objective in elevating SVR and reducing the drive to right-to-left shunting is to reinstate adequate coronary perfusion pressure. Achieving this goal increases the contractility of the systemic ventricle, ultimately supporting diuresis, lowering ventricular end-diastolic pressure, and preventing further myocardial damage. Vasopressors such as norepinephrine, phenylephrine, or vasopressin can all be used to increase SVR, thereby enhancing aortic root pressure. The success of this approach may vary among patients, and any intervention should be evaluated for its effects on arterial saturation.

Just as important is maintaining efforts to lower PVR. It is advisable to continue pulmonary vasodilators that patients have been prescribed as part of their standard therapy despite their association with systemic vasodilation and reduced SVR. As mentioned previously, this effect can be counterbalanced by adding vasopressors. Since introducing a new pulmonary vasodilator in hypotension, inhaled pulmonary vasodilators can be used more safely. These include inhaled agents such as nitric oxide, iloprost, epoprostenol, and treprostinil.

- *Augment cardiac output*

Both should be considered because cardiac output is the product of heart rate and stroke volume. Ensuring an appropriate sinus rhythm or sinus tachycardia plays a role in stabilizing a patient with cyanosis. Antiarrhythmic agents, cardioversion, or pacing can all be used when necessary. Tachyarrhythmias can trigger or result from ADHF. Control of a rapid ventricular rate and cardioversion is essential when tachyarrhythmias occur. To ensure safety during sedation and following cardioversion, we recommend sedation be instigated slowly and minimized. Even light sedation, if it results in a drop in arterial blood pressure, can drop SVR to catastrophic levels. Transvenous pacers increase the risk of systemic thromboembolic events and are best avoided.[27] When needed, the patient should be anticoagulated.

The utilization of inotropic agents should be reserved for patients with a low cardiac output unrelated to hypovolemia, in conjunction with signs of end-organ hypoperfusion, and only for a short duration. This cautious approach is taken because inotropes can reduce SVR, potentially leading to an imbalance between SVR and PVR, as warned above. Furthermore, inotropes may induce tachycardia, particularly in patients with concurrent atrial fibrillation, tachyarrhythmias, myocardial ischemia, and an associated increase in mortality.[28]

It is essential to note that inotropic agents can also elevate myocardial oxygen demand, as previously discussed. Patients with cyanotic CHD have limited capacity to increase their oxygen delivery, which is why the lowest effective dose should be used to avoid paradoxically exacerbating myocardial function and worsening the overall problem.

Hemodynamic Considerations: Decongestion and Preload Optimization

Initiating decongestive management with diuretic therapy to address volume overload should be used when appropriate but only after a comprehensive assessment. Recall that certain triggers of ADHF may not necessarily be associated with hypervolemia, such as sepsis, anemia, or reduced PBF or alveolar gas exchange. In such instances, intravenous diuresis could exacerbate heart failure symptoms. It is also imperative to exercise caution to prevent hyperviscosity resulting from hemoconcentration from excessive diuretic use. However, when needed, loop diuretics and diuretic augmentation can be considered as they would in a standard heart failure patient.

Decrease Metabolic Needs

Whatever can be done to minimize the oxygen consumption demands of the body, although still allowing crucial end-organ function to continue, might be worthwhile when oxygen delivery is compromised. Such strategies could include light sedation, pain management, avoiding excessive ambulation, avoiding large meals, ensuring euthyroid states, and so forth.

Mechanical Ventilation

Personnel within a standard health-care system often react quickly to low oxygen saturations with supplemental oxygen followed by noninvasive positive pressure ventilation. Many patients with cyanosis can share their experiences of visiting emergency departments and being offered such therapies immediately yet erroneously when at their baseline. Mechanical ventilatory assistance should be reserved for situations where the lung parenchyma or chest wall mechanics are compromised and not used solely to correct a low oxygen saturation.

Patients experiencing respiratory distress, characterized by a respiratory rate exceeding 25 breaths per minute, an SaO_2 level significantly lower than baseline, or respiratory acidosis on blood gas, can be started on noninvasive mechanical ventilation (bilevel positive airway pressure

[BiPAP]), provided their mental status is suitable. This approach is advised to minimize the need for mechanical ventilation and endotracheal intubation whenever feasible.

While at times necessary, endotracheal intubation should only be offered as a last resort, only for compromised pulmonary issues, including hemoptysis, and after discussing with the patient and family members. This includes addressing the potential risks of severe desaturation and hypotension during the intubation process, among other risks. Recall that many patients have anticipated their clinical demise during many decades and may opt against escalating treatment in favor of comfort measures.

Despite the associated risks, mechanical ventilation becomes necessary when patients become severely and newly hypercapnic or experience respiratory distress to avoid the imbalance between SVR and PVR. The main objectives of mechanical ventilation are to maintain efficient gas exchange, reduce breathing workload, and enhance patient comfort. However, because ventilation comes with obligatory sedation, an inherent SVR lowering can be detrimental, as discussed above.

The ideal mechanical ventilation strategy should alleviate respiratory distress by lessening excessive respiratory burden while preserving an appropriate level of spontaneous effort (preventing atrophy of the diaphragm and respiratory muscles) and ensuring harmonious interaction between the patient and the ventilator. Achieving this balance can be delicate, especially in the context of chronic hypoxemia. The mismatch between the patient's needs and the level of support provided by the machine can lead to dyssynchrony, resulting in challenges during weaning from ventilation, extended periods of mechanical ventilation, and decreased survival rates among adults with cyanotic CHD.[29–32]

Other considerations during the mechanical ventilation of patients with cyanotic CHD include the avoidance of high tidal volumes, given that these patients sometimes experience chronic CO_2 retention. Significantly, increased tidal volumes could suppress spontaneous ventilation and potentially lead to the diaphragm and respiratory muscle atrophy. Similarly, the primary goal during mechanical ventilation should not be to normalize oxygen saturation or CO_2 levels but to maintain them close to the patient's baseline.

Other Inpatient Care Issues

- *The role of pulmonary artery catheters*

PA catheters offer physiologically guided management by assessing pressure, cardiac output, and vascular resistance, aiding health-care providers in adjusting preload, afterload, and contractility. However, the clinical utility of PA catheters is constrained in patients with cyanotic CHD, even in scenarios involving low cardiac output and organ hypoperfusion. First, measuring PVR and SVR does not mandate PA pressure measurements, as the relative resistances of pulmonary and systemic circulations can be inferred through systemic oxygen saturation, assessable via pulse oximetry. Second, obtaining precise PVR and SVR measurements is more challenging than with PA catheters, given residual shunting and complex anatomic and physiologic factors. Third, there is a notable risk of PA rupture, especially in the presence of pulmonary hypertension and coagulation dysfunction. Consequently, we strongly discourage the use of PA catheters as a guide for managing patients with unrepaired or partially repaired cyanotic CHD.

- *Intravenous filters*

In principle, air and particulate matter have the potential to cause systemic embolization in individuals with right-to-left shunting. Consequently, guidelines for adult CHD recommend using air/particulate filters on all intravenous access lines to prevent the passage of air or particulate matter into the systemic circulation.[33] Yet the standard of care should include de-airing all lines to prevent the introduction of air or particulate matter, regardless of the presence of a filter.

- *Deep vein thrombosis prophylaxis*

It is advisable to use low-molecular-weight heparin for thromboembolism prevention in hospitalized patients with cyanosis and ADHF, provided they are not already receiving anticoagulation therapy and have no contraindications to anticoagulation. This approach helps reduce the risk of deep vein thrombosis and subsequent pulmonary and systemic embolism, including embolic stroke. Despite the presence of coagulation factor abnormalities in adults with cyanotic CHD, we believe that the advantages of thromboembolism prophylaxis outweigh the potential risks.

Case Outcome: The patient's oxygen delivery was supported with supplemental oxygen, iron, and occasional red blood cell transfusions to maintain a sufficient elevation of his hemoglobin. Additional increases in oxygen supplementation typically yielded no additional improvement. He was started on inhaled iloprost as well as continuing sildenafil and macitentan. With periods of significant desaturation, he was given norepinephrine infusion, titrated to blood pressure of greater than 130 systolic, and oxygen saturation

greater than 80%. He developed atrial fibrillation, and hence he was cardioverted and given amiodarone.

After 3 weeks of gradual but stalling progress, a tracheostomy was performed to avoid excessive ongoing sedation. His viral pneumonia improved. However, his neuromuscular status weakened, with significant muscle atrophy despite adequate ongoing nutrition. Systemic blood pressure often remained low. He failed several spontaneous breathing trials due to low tidal volumes.

During the ensuing months, many attempts were made to encourage the patient to rehabilitate his muscle groups to increase strength. Still, language and understanding were complex, given his Down syndrome and tracheostomy. After 9 months in the hospital with daily attempts to improve his condition and numerous discussions with family members about his care goals, he had failed to progress. He developed rapid atrial arrhythmia intractable to any therapy. A few days later, he suddenly became pulseless with agonal beats and cardiovascular collapse.

MANAGEMENT OF CHRONIC HEART FAILURE IN CYANOSIS

Case presentation: A 27-year-old woman with a double outlet right ventricle underwent PA banding in infancy but additional repair was never undertaken. For most of her life, she was functional with "balanced" circulation and oxygen saturation of 88%. She did not feel limited and worked as a cashier for many years. Gradually, however, her stamina worsened. She developed gout, a brain abscess that was drained, severe menorrhagia, and iron deficiency. In the clinic, she had a loud systolic murmur. Oxygen saturation was 72% at rest. Her hemoglobin was 14 g/dL, and her transferrin saturation (TSAT) was 12%.

Individuals with cyanotic CHD exhibit both structural and functional abnormalities that relate to chronic shunting and relative hypoxia gradually over time, inevitably leading to chronic cardiovascular failure. Managing heart failure is, therefore, most often done in the outpatient setting. There is a wide heterogeneity of underlying anatomic and surgical repair differences and a wide spectrum of potential heart failure causes.[34] For most, attempts at definitive treatment to separate the 2 circulations carry unacceptably high mortality risks due to many factors, including chronic multiorgan dysfunction and risks of general anesthesia. At times, however, intervention may be worth the risk.

The general goals of oxygen delivery and optimization discussed earlier are also applicable for chronic management of failing cyanosis, although used differently outside of a hospital setting. Strategies that can be considered, which may differ based on the presence or absence of a systolic ejection murmur, are discussed as follows.

Improve Pulmonary Blood Flow

The universal strategy to assist a struggling cyanotic is to augment effective PBF. This goal differs significantly when there is an anatomic obstruction in pulmonary flow versus when there is none. With a murmur, there should be discussion around ways to augment PBF. This might mean a central or peripheral shunt placed operatively.

When there is no murmur, such as with ES, blood flow augmentation requires pulmonary vasodilators. Pulmonary vasodilators (eg, endothelin receptor antagonists, phosphodiesterase inhibitors, and prostanoids) have demonstrated favorable effects, which are beyond the scope of this review.

Support Hemoglobin and Iron Stores

Iron deficiency is a common issue in patients with cyanosis, primarily due to the depletion of iron stores caused by increased demand or chronic bleeding. Those with iron deficiency exhibit lower resting oxygen saturation, reduced hemoglobin levels, and a higher red blood cell count, while hematocrit levels remain consistent.[13]

There is a general trend toward macrocytosis. Therefore, mean corpuscular volume (MCV) is an inadequate screening tool for iron deficiency. We recommend using TSAT as a screening tool for iron deficiency because multiple heart failure trials have used this method.[35–37] Oral iron supplementation may be hindered by gastrointestinal side effects related to poor absorption and a longer "time to effect" than intravenous administration. Consequently, intravenous supplementation is sometimes preferred for patients with significantly low iron stores. Once iron stores are replenished, iron supplements should be discontinued, and a regular balanced diet should be encouraged.

Treating Myocardial Dysfunction

There is currently no definitive evidence to support the use of contemporary heart failure guideline-directed medical therapy (eg, angiotensin receptor/neprilysin inhibitor, beta-blocker) in patients with partially repaired or unrepaired cyanotic CHD. This lack of evidence is attributed to our limited understanding of the precise mechanisms of heart failure in these patients and the absence of studies demonstrating the benefits of such medical therapy.[28]

It is important to note that medical therapies designed to enhance heart function, whether in patients with reduced left ventricular systolic function or preserved left ventricular systolic function, typically aim to reduce SVR. However, in the case of patients with cyanotic CHD, lowering SVR may exacerbate right-to-left shunting, leading to deteriorating hypoxemia and hypotension. This can subsequently result in myocardial ischemia and a series of events that may ultimately lead to cardiogenic shock.

Oxygen Supplementation

Health-care providers need to exercise caution when considering oxygen therapy for patients with cyanotic CHD. These patients may have lung disease and compensatory respiratory alkalosis. Administering oxygen to achieve normal oxygen saturation levels may inhibit the patient's respiratory drive.[17] Oxygen supplementation is a vital therapeutic approach for managing cyanosis because it enhances oxygen delivery. The focus should be on alleviating symptoms associated with cyanosis rather than fixating on precise oxygen saturation targets.[38]

Anticoagulation Role

The balance between hemorrhage and thromboembolism as causes of death among patients with cyanosis with CHD strongly leans toward thromboembolism. Therefore, the consideration of anticoagulation in patients with cyanotic CHD is advisable.[18] However, the German National CHD Registry reported that 17.6% of patients with ES received anticoagulants, whereas 23.5% were administered aspirin. Interestingly, this did not affect survival, as indicated by the registry data.[39] Consequently, it is crucial to weigh the risks and benefits of anticoagulation in individual patients with coagulopathy, considering the potential risk of major hemorrhage.

Current European adults with CHD guidelines state that anticoagulation in ES should be offered for atrial arrhythmias and in the presence of PA thrombus or embolism in patients at low risk of bleeding.[40,41]

Role of Device Therapy

Intracardiac and subcutaneous defibrillators (ICD and Sub-Q defibrillators) are high-intensity interventions that may extend life span without necessarily improving the quality of life. Although both devices can save lives by terminating lethal arrhythmias, they do not enhance cardiac function or alleviate heart failure symptoms. Sub-Q defibrillators are preferred over ICDs due to a lower risk of systemic embolization. Although the use of Sub-Q defibrillators for secondary prevention is widely accepted, there is no consensus on their use for primary prevention. Patients with severe systemic ventricle dysfunction, unexplained syncope, or nonsustained VT may be suitable candidates for Sub-Q defibrillator placement. It is crucial to consider the potential drawbacks, such as the risk of inappropriate shocks, increased hospitalization risk, potential impact on quality of life, and a higher likelihood of death from pump failure.[42] Therefore, we recommend shared decision-making regarding Sub-Q defibrillator placement, especially for patients with advanced disease who are not candidates for heart/lung transplants.

The Clinical Utility of Wearable Biosensors

The effectiveness of wearable biosensors in reducing hospitalizations due to heart failure remains uncertain among adults with cyanotic CHD because the conventional definition of heart failure in adults may not apply to this population because it encompasses both cardiogenic or pulmonary congestion and reduced tissue oxygen delivery.[7] Consequently, wearable sensors for hemodynamic assessment may not necessarily reduce heart failure hospitalizations or contribute significantly to medical decision-making. Nevertheless, wearable biosensors offer diverse physiologic measurements that hold clinical value for adults with cyanotic CHD.[43]

The remote monitoring and measurement of oxygen saturation, heart rate, heart rate variability, blood pressure, and step count using various wearable biosensors can effectively identify pattern changes as early indicators of adverse clinical events. Given the significance of oxygen saturation, heart rate, and blood pressure as vital signs in this population, analyzing these data can serve as a valuable starting point for detecting the initial stages of ADHF. This approach encourages clinicians to optimize oxygen delivery to tissues in a timely manner.[43]

Case Outcome

To enhance her functional capacity, she underwent systemic-to-pulmonary artery shunt procedures to optimize effective PBF. Given a prominent murmur and elevated gradients across the PA, shunt placement was the most effective means of enhancing effective PBF rather than using pulmonary vasodilators. She received intravenous iron supplementation in response to iron deficiency anemia, improving her functional capacity. To address menorrhagia, a Mirena intrauterine device was inserted. As a result, her oxygen saturation returned to her baseline in the high 80s, and her functional capacity reverted to baseline levels, enabling her to resume work.

MANAGEMENT OF END-STAGE CYANOTIC HEART FAILURE
Heart Transplant and Mechanical Circulatory Support Considerations

Mechanical circulatory support or extracorporeal membrane oxygenation (ECMO) is primarily suitable for addressing acute and reversible causes, such as pneumonia. When individuals experience a decline in functional ability despite pharmacologic treatment of pulmonary arterial hypertension, consideration should be given to heart-lung transplantation. However, standardized indications for such therapies in adults with cyanotic CHD (CHD) are currently lacking.

It is important to note that the rate of heart or heart-lung transplantation is relatively lower among adults with CHD (comprising 3% of all heart transplants) compared with the non-CHD population.[44,45] Patients with ES have a similarly low rate of heart-lung or lung transplants (9%), and there is a higher mortality rate among those late on the transplant waiting list.[46–49]

This leads to the question of who would benefit from a heart/lung transplant and when the ideal time for referral for such a procedure would be among adults with partially repaired or unrepaired cyanotic CHD. The 1-year mortality rate on the heart transplant waiting list is higher for adults with CHD compared with those without (24% vs 15%).[50–52] This suggests that referral for a heart-lung transplant typically occurs late in the disease process. This delay may be due to the limited number of centers capable of performing heart-lung transplants for patients with CHD with complex anatomy, multiple interventional procedures, advanced age, and multiorgan dysfunction, which are often prevalent and concerning characteristics.[53]

A recent study of patients with ES who underwent heart transplantation showed a median survival of 12 years after heart-lung transplant and low rates of common complications such as cardiac allograft vasculopathy, bronchiolitis obliterans syndrome, and renal failure requiring dialysis.[46] Therefore, identifying the appropriate patients with ES who will benefit from transplantation is paramount.

It remains uncertain whether scoring systems developed to predict mortality among adults with pulmonary arterial hypertension can also be used to predict mortality and prompt early referral for heart-lung transplants among adults with cyanotic CHD, particularly the REVEAL score.[54,55]

In terms of noninvasive predictors of mortality with conventional therapy among adults with cyanotic CHD who may benefit from early referral for heart-lung transplant, factors such as increasing age, ASD, decreased oxygen saturation, lack of sinus rhythm, and the presence of pericardial effusion is considered significant.[49] In cases where medical treatment using pulmonary vasodilators provides a similar survival benefit to a heart-lung transplant, it may be a preferred option.

It is important to highlight that the United Network for Organ Sharing (UNOS) does not acknowledge deteriorating chronic cyanosis unresponsive to interventions aimed at improving effective PBF and instances of hemoptysis in adults with CHD as qualifying indications for heart-lung transplantation. Given the elevated risk of adverse cardiac events associated with both worsening cyanosis and hemoptysis, the progression of cyanosis or occurrences of hemoptysis should be considered as a criterion for inclusion in heart-lung transplantation listings.[56]

For adults with cyanotic CHD admitted for ADHF, ECMO could be considered as a bridge to lung transplantation or recovery, particularly in treatment-naive or nonoptimized patients. However, adults with cyanotic CHD are unlikely to benefit from venoarterial ECMO alone because these patients often experience concurrent lung failure. In such cases, veno-arterial-venous ECMO is indicated.

In the United States, the matching process for heart-lung transplants is primarily based on the heart allocation match list rather than the lung allocation match list. UNOS permits a higher listing on the heart allocation list following the submission of an exception request by the transplant center.

A heart-lung transplant is considered a high-intensity intervention that can enhance both quantity and quality of life. Before assuming this option, there should be direct discussions with the patient involving informed consent and shared decision-making regarding overall care goals, preferences, and prognosis, supported by evidence-based medical information.

Palliative Care and Hospice

The definition of stage D heart failure provided by the American Heart Association/American College of Cardiology/European Society of Cardiology cannot be directly applied to adults with cyanotic CHD. This definition primarily focuses on end-stage cardiomyopathy and does not consider the decreased oxygen delivery issues or the adaptations that sometimes allow for ongoing survival in CHD.[28,57] Cyanotic CHD-related heart failure is so much more than cardiac function.

Yet identifying the later stage of their illness is still important. They have been living with the belief that their death is imminent throughout their lives. One of the challenges in addressing end-of-life care is that most individuals were initially told that they might not survive to adulthood and have already survived well beyond expectations. Therefore, accurate prognostication is difficult and should be acknowledged. As always, an approach focused on symptom management without necessarily postponing death is essential. However, the prognosis is improving, with more and safer interventional options and pulmonary vasodilators.[58] Although it is often advisable to include palliative care clinicians who have received comprehensive training in managing refractory symptoms and facilitating complex care planning for life-threatening illnesses, such a team needs instruction from an ACHD provider on the nature of cyanotic CHD and prognostic uncertainties.

When the end of life is expected, hospice can be pursued after 2 providers that the patient's life expectancy is 6 months or less. Given that most patients with cyanotic CHD have already outlived multiple expectations of their longevity by years or even decades, making such a declaration may seem arbitrary. Patients have already adapted to their limitations and may prefer to stay home. However, when needed, hospice care can provide respite and additional comfort. Hospice care offers several advantages to patients and their families, including home visits, respite care, the provision of medications and durable medical equipment, and access to a nurse who can guide urgent symptom management. The patient must be willing to forgo conventional medical services aimed at curing the underlying terminal diagnosis. However, it is often advisable to continue using oral pulmonary vasodilators because they relieve symptoms and help reduce hypoxia. Transitioning from intravenous and inhaled pulmonary vasodilators to their oral forms simplifies administration and is appropriate, depending on the policies of individual hospice agencies.[59] In cases where patients live beyond the 6-month window, they can often continue receiving hospice benefits if their poor prognosis persists.

SUMMARY

CHD is an uncommon condition because, in most cases of CHD, biventricular or single ventricle repair is feasible. However, developing a comprehensive understanding of the physiology of unrepaired or partially repaired cyanotic CHD is crucial. This knowledge is essential for effectively addressing heart failure symptoms, managing associated comorbidities, and handling episodes of acute heart failure exacerbation.

The management of heart failure in adults with cyanotic CHD aims to maximize SOT. This is typically achieved by increasing cardiac output, optimizing oxygen-carrying capacity, and maintaining an appropriate hemoglobin level.

CLINICS CARE POINTS

- Cyanotic CHD can be classified anatomically, considering the presence of PBF obstruction, or physiologically, based on total, systemic, and effective pulmonary flow measurements.

- Heart failure in individuals with cyanotic CHD is distinctive in that it involves both cardiomyopathy and reduced oxygen delivery to the tissues.

- The primary objective in managing patients with cyanotic CHD should be to enhance their SOT (oxygen delivery capacity).

DISCLOSURE

The authors have nothing to disclose.

REFERENCES

1. van der Linde D, Konings EE, Slager MA, et al. Birth prevalence of congenital heart disease worldwide: a systematic review and meta-analysis. J Am Coll Cardiol 2011;58:2241–7.
2. Hoffman JI, Kaplan S. The incidence of congenital heart disease. J Am Coll Cardiol 2002;39:1890–900.
3. Warnes CA, Liberthson R, Danielson GK, et al. Task force 1: the changing profile of congenital heart disease in adult life. J Am Coll Cardiol 2001;37:1170–5.
4. Norozi K, Wessel A, Alpers V, et al. Incidence and risk distribution of heart failure in adolescents and adults with congenital heart disease after cardiac surgery. Am J Cardiol 2006;97:1238–43.
5. Piran S, Veldtman G, Siu S, et al. Heart failure and ventricular dysfunction in patients with single or systemic right ventricles. Circulation 2002;105:1189–94.
6. Duffels MG, Engelfriet PM, Berger RM, et al. Pulmonary arterial hypertension in congenital heart disease: an epidemiologic perspective from a Dutch registry. Int J Cardiol 2007;120:198–204.
7. Bozkurt B, Coats AJ, Tsutsui H, et al. Universal Definition and Classification of Heart Failure: A Report of the Heart Failure Society of America, Heart Failure Association of the European Society of Cardiology, Japanese Heart Failure Society and Writing Committee of the Universal Definition of Heart Failure. J Card Fail 2021;27:387–413.
8. Leach RM, Treacher DF. The pulmonary physician in critical care • 2: Oxygen delivery and consumption in the critically ill. Thorax 2002;57:170–7.
9. Martin L, Khalil H. How much reduced hemoglobin is necessary to generate central cyanosis? Chest 1990;97:182–5.
10. Broberg CS, Jayaweera AR, Diller GP, et al. Seeking optimal relation between oxygen saturation and hemoglobin concentration in adults with cyanosis from congenital heart disease. Am J Cardiol 2011; 107:595–9.
11. Adelman DM, Maltepe E, Simon MC. Multilineage embryonic hematopoiesis requires hypoxic ARNT activity. Genes Dev 1999;13:2478–83.
12. Yamashita T, Ohneda O, Sakiyama A, et al. The microenvironment for erythropoiesis is regulated by HIF-2alpha through VCAM-1 in endothelial cells. Blood 2008;112:1482–92.
13. Broberg CS, Bax BE, Okonko DO, et al. Blood viscosity and its relationship to iron deficiency, symptoms, and exercise capacity in adults with cyanotic congenital heart disease. J Am Coll Cardiol 2006;48:356–65.
14. Connolly DT, Olander JV, Heuvelman D, et al. Human vascular permeability factor. Isolation from U937 cells. J Biol Chem 1989;264:20017–24.
15. Liu Y, Cox SR, Morita T, et al. Hypoxia Regulates Vascular Endothelial Growth Factor Gene Expression in Endothelial Cells. Circ Res 1995;77:638–43.
16. Broberg CS, Ujita M, Prasad S, et al. Pulmonary arterial thrombosis in eisenmenger syndrome is associated with biventricular dysfunction and decreased pulmonary flow velocity. J Am Coll Cardiol 2007;50:634–42.
17. Broberg CS, Van Woerkom RC, Swallow E, et al. Lung function and gas exchange in Eisenmenger syndrome and their impact on exercise capacity and survival. Int J Cardiol 2014;171:73–7.
18. Hjortshøj CMS, Kempny A, Jensen AS, et al. Past and current cause-specific mortality in Eisenmenger syndrome. Eur Heart J 2017;38:2060–7.
19. Jensen AS, Johansson PI, Bochsen L, et al. Fibrinogen function is impaired in whole blood from patients with cyanotic congenital heart disease. Int J Cardiol 2013;167:2210–4.
20. Westbury SK, Lee K, Reilly-Stitt C, et al. High haematocrit in cyanotic congenital heart disease affects how fibrinogen activity is determined by rotational thromboelastometry. Thromb Res 2013;132:e145–51.
21. Henriksson P, Varendh G, Lundstrom NR. Haemostatic defects in cyanotic congenital heart disease. Br Heart J 1979;41:23–7.
22. Diller GP, Alonso-Gonzalez R, Kempny A, et al. B-type natriuretic peptide concentrations in contemporary

Eisenmenger syndrome patients: predictive value and response to disease targeting therapy. Heart 2012;98:736–42.

23. Reardon LC, Williams RJ, Houser LS, et al. Usefulness of serum brain natriuretic peptide to predict adverse events in patients with the Eisenmenger syndrome. Am J Cardiol 2012;110:1523–6.

24. Daliento L, Somerville J, Presbitero P, et al. Eisenmenger syndrome. Factors relating to deterioration and death. Eur Heart J 1998;19:1845–55.

25. Turgeman A, McRae HL, Cahill C, et al. Impact of RBC Transfusion on Peripheral Capillary Oxygen Saturation and Partial Pressure of Arterial Oxygen. Am J Clin Pathol 2021;156:149–54.

26. Ammash N, Warnes CA. Cerebrovascular events in adult patients with cyanotic congenital heart disease. J Am Coll Cardiol 1996;28:768–72.

27. Khairy P, Landzberg MJ, Gatzoulis MA, et al. Transvenous Pacing Leads and Systemic Thromboemboli in Patients With Intracardiac Shunts. Circulation 2006;113:2391–7.

28. Heidenreich PA, Bozkurt B, Aguilar D, et al. AHA/ACC/HFSA Guideline for the Management of Heart Failure: A Report of the American College of Cardiology/American Heart Association Joint Committee on Clinical Practice Guidelines. Circulation 2022;145:e895–1032.

29. Chao DC, Scheinhorn DJ, Stearn-Hassenpflug M. Patient-ventilator trigger asynchrony in prolonged mechanical ventilation. Chest 1997;112:1592–9.

30. Thille AW, Rodriguez P, Cabello B, et al. Patient-ventilator asynchrony during assisted mechanical ventilation. Intensive Care Med 2006;32:1515–22.

31. de Wit M, Miller KB, Green DA, et al. Ineffective triggering predicts increased duration of mechanical ventilation. Crit Care Med 2009;37:2740–5.

32. Vaporidi K, Babalis D, Chytas A, et al. Clusters of ineffective efforts during mechanical ventilation: impact on outcome. Intensive Care Med 2017;43:184–91.

33. Stout KK, Daniels CJ, Aboulhosn JA, et al. 2018 AHA/ACC Guideline for the Management of Adults With Congenital Heart Disease: A Report of the American College of Cardiology/American Heart Association Task Force on Clinical Practice Guidelines. Circulation 2019;139:e698–800.

34. Stout KK, Broberg CS, Book WM, et al. Chronic Heart Failure in Congenital Heart Disease. Circulation 2016;133:770–801.

35. Mentz RJ, Garg J, Rockhold FW, et al. Ferric Carboxymaltose in Heart Failure with Iron Deficiency. N Engl J Med 2023;389:975–86.

36. Kalra PR, Cleland JGF, Petrie MC, et al. Intravenous ferric derisomaltose in patients with heart failure and iron deficiency in the UK (IRONMAN): an investigator-initiated, prospective, randomised, open-label, blinded-endpoint trial. Lancet 2022;400:2199–209. https://doi.org/10.1016/s0140-6736(22)02083-9.

37. Ponikowski P, Kirwan BA, Anker SD, et al. Ferric carboxymaltose for iron deficiency at discharge after acute heart failure: a multicentre, double-blind, randomised, controlled trial. Lancet 2020;396:1895–904.

38. Berman W Jr, Wood SC, Yabek SM, et al. Systemic oxygen transport in patients with congenital heart disease. Circulation 1987;75:360–8.

39. Diller G-P, Körten M-A, Bauer UM, et al. Current therapy and outcome of Eisenmenger syndrome: data of the German National Register for congenital heart defects. Eur Heart J 2016;37:1449–55.

40. Baumgartner H, De Backer J, Babu-Narayan SV, et al. 2020 ESC Guidelines for the management of adult congenital heart disease: the Task Force for the management of adult congenital heart disease of the European Society of Cardiology (ESC). Endorsed by: Association for European Paediatric and Congenital Cardiology (AEPC), International Society for Adult Congenital Heart Disease (ISACHD). Eur Heart J 2021;42:563–645.

41. Sandoval Zarate J, Jerjes-Sanchez C, Ramirez-Rivera A, et al. Mexican registry of pulmonary hypertension: REMEHIP. Arch Cardiol Mex 2017;87:13–7.

42. McDonagh TA, Metra M, Adamo M, et al. Corrigendum to: 2021 ESC Guidelines for the diagnosis and treatment of acute and chronic heart failure: Developed by the Task Force for the diagnosis and treatment of acute and chronic heart failure of the European Society of Cardiology (ESC) With the special contribution of the Heart Failure Association (HFA) of the ESC. Eur Heart J 2021;42:4901.

43. Tandon A, Nguyen HH, Avula S, et al. Wearable Biosensors in Congenital Heart Disease. JACC (J Am Coll Cardiol): Advances 2023;2:100267.

44. Goldberg SW, Fisher SA, Wehman B, et al. Adults with congenital heart disease and heart transplantation: optimizing outcomes. J Heart Lung Transplant 2014;33:873–7.

45. Crossland DS, Jansen K, Parry G, et al. Outcome following heart transplant assessment in adults with congenital heart disease. Heart 2019;105:1741–7.

46. Hjortshøj CS, Gilljam T, Dellgren G, et al. Outcome after heart–lung or lung transplantation in patients with Eisenmenger syndrome. Heart 2020;106:127–32.

47. Farber HW, Miller DP, Poms AD, et al. Five-Year outcomes of patients enrolled in the REVEAL Registry. Chest 2015;148:1043–54.

48. Barst RJ, Ivy DD, Foreman AJ, et al. Four- and seven-year outcomes of patients with congenital heart disease-associated pulmonary arterial hypertension (from the REVEAL Registry). Am J Cardiol 2014;113:147–55.

49. Kempny A, Hjortshøj CS, Gu H, et al. Predictors of Death in Contemporary Adult Patients With Eisenmenger Syndrome: A Multicenter Study. Circulation 2017;135:1432–40.

50. Alshawabkeh LI, Hu N, Carter KD, et al. Wait-List Outcomes for Adults With Congenital Heart Disease Listed for Heart Transplantation in the U.S. J Am Coll Cardiol 2016;68:908–17.

51. Hsich EM, Rogers JG, McNamara DM, et al. Does Survival on the Heart Transplant Waiting List Depend on the Underlying Heart Disease? JACC Heart Fail 2016;4:689–97.

52. Blackstone EH, Rajeswaran J, Cruz VB, et al. Continuously Updated Estimation of Heart Transplant Waitlist Mortality. J Am Coll Cardiol 2018;72:650–9.

53. Dolgner SJ, Nguyen VP, Krieger EV, et al. Long-term adult congenital heart disease survival after heart transplantation: A restricted mean survival time analysis. J Heart Lung Transplant 2021;40:698–706.

54. Benza RL, Miller DP, Barst RJ, et al. An evaluation of long-term survival from time of diagnosis in pulmonary arterial hypertension from the REVEAL Registry. Chest 2012;142:448–56.

55. Humbert M, Kovacs G, Hoeper MM, et al. ESC/ERS Guidelines for the diagnosis and treatment of pulmonary hypertension: Developed by the task force for the diagnosis and treatment of pulmonary hypertension of the European Society of Cardiology (ESC) and the European Respiratory Society (ERS). Endorsed by the International Society for Heart and Lung Transplantation (ISHLT) and the European Reference Network on rare respiratory diseases (ERN-LUNG). Eur Heart J 2022;43:3618–731.

56. Lubert AM, Cedars A, Almond CS, et al. Considerations for Advanced Heart Failure Consultation in Individuals With Fontan Circulation: Recommendations From ACTION. Circulation: Heart Fail 2023;16:e010123.

57. Crespo-Leiro MG, Metra M, Lund LH, et al. Advanced heart failure: a position statement of the Heart Failure Association of the European Society of Cardiology. Eur J Heart Fail 2018;20:1505–35.

58. Hou Y, Wen L, Shu T, et al. Efficacy and safety of pulmonary vasodilators in the patients with Eisenmenger syndrome: a meta-analysis of randomized controlled trials. Pulm Circ 2021;11. 20458940211015823.

59. Lum HD, Horney C, Koets D, et al. Availability of Heart Failure Medications in Hospice Care. Am J Hosp Palliat Care 2016;33:924–8.

Palliative Care in Adult Congenital Heart Disease– Associated Advanced Heart Disease

Michael J. Landzberg, MD[a,b,c,*]

KEYWORDS

- Suffering • Palliative care • Communication • Adult congenital heart disease
- Advanced heart disease • Heart failure

KEY POINTS

- Palliative care (PC) is nearly universally practiced as an attempt to mitigate an individual's suffering via mechanisms and strategies that take into account the composite of that person's physical, psychological, social, and spiritual stressors and influences.
- Primary medical issues and so-called "disease-targeting therapies" (which remain under the guidance and care of primary disease–targeting clinicians, for the sake of this article, namely adult congenital heart disease or advanced heart disease clinicians) often bring an individual to a PC clinician's attention due to a heightening of symptoms, medical adversities, or uncertainties in medical outcomes.
- Palliative care is an iterative and longitudinal process (assessing patient priorities, values, goals and sense of intolerable occurrences, and aligning such with care plans) with various components changing over an individual's lifetime

INTRODUCTION

Palliative care (PC) is nearly universally practiced as an attempt to mitigate an individual's suffering via mechanisms and strategies that take into account the composite of that persons' physical, psychological, social, and spiritual (PPSS) stressors and influences (**Fig. 1**). Primary medical issues and so-called "disease-targeting therapies" (which remain under the guidance and care of primary disease–targeting clinicians, for the sake of this article, namely adult congenital heart disease [ACHD], or advanced heart disease [AHD] clinicians) often bring an individual to a PC clinician's attention due to a heightening of symptoms, medical adversities, or uncertainties in medical

outcomes. The PC consulting clinician or team is tasked to assist the primary team in better understanding patient (and supporting social structure) priorities, hopes and values, clarifying and optimizing medical communication between patients and supports and medical teams, and aligning proposed disease-targeting care plans with patient goals. To optimize outcomes, members within the PC team may help to assess and build relevant strengths and supports from within the unique and constantly evolving PPSS fabric that makes up the particular individual and personal narrative.

To the non-PC clinician, the earlier sentinel paragraph may appear to be a "mouthful of

a Boston Adult Congenital Heart (BACH) Group, Heart Pal Team; b Department of Cardiology, Brigham and Women's Hospital, Boston Children's Hospital, Harvard Medical School, 300 Longwood Avenue, Boston, MA 02115, USA; c Department of Psychosocial Oncology and Palliative Care, Dana Farber Cancer Institute
* Corresponding author. BACH Group, Department of Cardiology, BWH and Boston Children's Hospital, 300 Longwood Avenue, Boston, MA 02115.
E-mail address: Mike.Landzberg@cardio.chboston.org

Heart Failure Clin 20 (2024) 237–243
https://doi.org/10.1016/j.hfc.2023.12.005
1551-7136/24/© 2023 Elsevier Inc. All rights reserved.

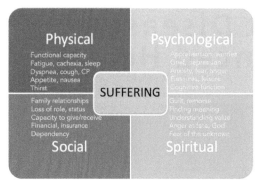

Fig. 1. A schema of some of the physical, psychological, social and spiritual contributors to suffering.

intangible theoretics." To place this into meaningful context, this article will present several circumstances not uncommon to the ACHD and AHD clinician (the presenting medical specifics of which are not the focus of the ensuing discussion), and will demonstrate the role that a PC clinician or team can have, with supportive data where such exist. A sense of need for further embedding of PC systems within ACHD teams will likely develop in the reader, along with recognition of gaps in the validation of such a "need".

As a prologue, PC practice appears relevant to the overlap between ACHD and AHD because

a. Such patients carry a high burden of cardiac and noncardiac symptomatology, with attendant suffering.[1] A commonly used phrase in our care team is that "ACHD physiologically and clinically are 20 to 30 years older than their stated ages," as symptom burden and both cardiovascular and noncardiovascular morbid and mortal risks (functional capacity, atrial arrhythmia, stroke, chronic kidney disease, systemic and pulmonary vascular disease, heart failure with reduced ejection fraction, heart failure with preserved ejection fraction (HFpEF), cancer risk), as well as resource and hospital resource utilization far exceed that for age-matched and gender-matched controls, typically to levels of others decades older than patient age.

b. With both anatomic and physiologic contributors to such symptom burden, there are (i) frequent transitions in care (home to hospital, pharmacologic changes, mechanical interventions, and so forth) and (ii) predictable and less predictable trajectories of decline.[2,3]

c. PPSS contributors to both suffering and coping appear highly complex, acknowledging (i) effects of early childhood hypoxia and surgery, as well as congenital syndromes, on cognitive and relational processing, (ii) lifelong

uncertainty of timing and outcomes of repeat interventions, (iii) competing sense of invincibility and vulnerability, by the patient, family, and clinical teams, (iv) common presence of compounded trauma and loss, and (v) multifactorial contributors to limitations in social and societal roles, as well as self-image.

Patient Scenario 1

You are called to see a 55-year-old man with D-loop transposition of the great arteries with intact ventricular septum, status post (s/p) atrial switch, in the setting of heart failure and VT storm, with intercostal nerve blocks in place. Past history includes pacemaker placed for sinus node dysfunction, intra-atrial reentrant tachycardia s/p ablation, and moderate-to-severe systemic right ventricular systolic dysfunction, with moderate-to-severe tricuspid regurgitation, chronic kidney disease-stage 3, liver fibrosis, and several recent hospitalizations for acute decompensated heart failure (ADHF) over the past year, including one several months ago for ventricular tachycardia (leading to the placement of implantable cardioverter defibrillator). As you sit down to begin your interview, the first question you are asked by the patient is, "*Doctor, do you believe in God?*"

Discussion: scenario 1

Numerous points for elaboration can be highlighted in this short vignette, describing an adult with congenital heart disease in his mid-50s, with multiple noncardiovascular comorbidities, recurrent hospitalizations for ADHF, and acute threat to survival of VT storm, who greets consulting staff with a question that appears seemingly impertinent to the process of the interview.

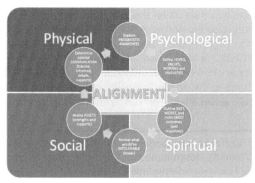

Fig. 2. The central role of a serious illness conversation in aligning care plans with patient goals of care for adult congenital heart disease with advanced heart disease.

- Serious illness conversations (SICs) and advanced care planning:

  Prior to review of SICs in the ACHD population, a general review of the nature of such interactions between health care clinicians and patients and their supports seems warranted (**Fig. 2**).

  Intrinsic to any therapeutic SIC is the very basic question of **how a patient prefers to communicate**, that is, (a) desire to have specific details, as contrasted to the "big picture," when it comes to medical discussions, (b) when important prognostic or diagnostic or therapeutic discussions arise, is there a wish for particular supports to be present, such as a health care proxy?

  Conversations by PC clinicians are facilitated by the use of **trauma-informed communication** principles, which hold several key components at their foundation: (i) asking permission to broach important questions or to share revelations, (ii) speaking in small aliquots, in direct and transparent fashion, and in cognitive age-appropriate and sociologically appropriate terminology, allowing for emotions to be expressed, and for accrual of supports or a "time-out", prior to reengagement.

  Such SIC often begin with an exploration of whether a patient has been made aware of current medical status, prognosis, and anticipated health trajectory (in a fashion relevant to the patient). Further inquiry extends questioning into that particular setting, including what would be most important, given these health facts, to this patient. What brings greatest joy and meaning? What would a "good outcome" and a "bad outcome" look like? What does the patient worry about the most? What possible outcomes, in particular, losses (eg, loss of function, image, role, experiences, meaning) would seem intolerable? What and who support this patient in medical decision-making and consequences of interventions? Has the patient contemplated what would happen if bad, or worst case, outcomes occurred?

  So often clinicians sense an imperative to define "limits to life-sustaining therapies, that is, LLST", and will ask the difficult (and subjectively biased) questions of, "Do you want your ribs cracked, or a breathing machine placed in you, if your heart was to stop?" In fact, such conversations place unrealistic burdens within a therapeutic clinician-patient relationship, which mandates that patients and families recognize and express their hopes, values, and priorities, and that clinicians translate such to the best of their abilities in their development of care plans. The finesse of a meaningful SIC allows a clinician to ultimately know what priorities are most important for a patient, and to make recommendations, and guide treatment plans, inclusive of LLST, to attempt to best protect priorities and avoid intolerable outcomes

  With particular regard to ACHD, data suggest that they, in fact, hope, and are willing, to have SICs early in their medical course, prior to their development of severe illness.[4–6] That being said, the occurrence and documentation of SICs in ACHD appear to be low, in part related to (a) the patient's lack of familiarity with, or sense of inappropriate timing for, such discussion, (b) hesitancy by ACHD clinicians to hold such SICs.[6–8]

- Clinicians are tempted to treat all questions literally. A PC clinician might reflect, "Did this patient truly mean, "Do I believe in God?," and if so, how should I answer that? How will my answer stay relevant to my therapeutic role?"

  In the absence of fullest clarity in medical understanding, PC clinicians tend to fall back to **certain basic communication tools or phrases**. During a medical interview, when uncertainty occurs and greater detail or exploration is desired, clinicians can trial the short phrase, "*Tell me more*", to which a greater, more detailed response often ensues. Similarly, when greater numbers of patient options, as part of a fuller response, may be assistive to the clinician, the short phrase,

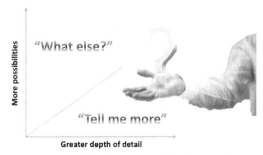

Fig. 3. Two simple phrases extend understanding.

"*What else*," may extend details in a fashion that aids greater understanding (**Fig. 3**).

- PC clinicians similarly find that "*normalizing*," that is, placing a response in a context in which other examples are given, may help a patient better express what they were having difficulty in self-expressing. For example, for this patient, the clinician might share, "When some people ask me about my faith and faith-practice, what they are really asking me is ...... (giving examples: (a) Am I dying?, (b) Do I have sufficient similarity to them to truly align with them?, or (c) What have I done to deserve all of the many adversities that are happening to me?)"

- The use of "*superlatives,*" that is, "most" or "least" within a probing question, can help coax a patient to share information that may at times feel more difficult for them to reveal. For example, the question, "What worries you, as you ask me about my belief in God?," may be met by a simple, "nothing," yet, when a PC clinician asks, "What worries you the **most**, as you ask me about my belief in God?," an expectation is left with the patient that worries exist, that it is safe to have such worries, and that it is OK to reflect and discuss them.

- *Existential concerns*: Whether it be (a) fears or the uncertainty of the unknowns in the trajectory of disease progression (or in the pathway and occurrence of end of life [EOL]), (b) sense of unfinished aspects of human or eternal relationships, or (c) questioning of why suffering exists as part of disease trajectory, and the natural sense of self-blame in such (eg, what did I do to deserve this punishment of suffering?), existential concerns run deep for persons with chronic illness, whether people have defined belief in faith-based practice or not.[9,10] PC clinicians and associated spiritual care consultants may feel skilled and experienced at "unpacking," therapeutically exploring and providing context and suggestions for adaptive coping for patients with such concerns; the benefits of systematic programming to address such existential worries on social-wellbeing and patient-centered preparedness for EOL, have been demonstrated.[11] For the ACHD or AHD clinician, "*naming*" the concern, in and of itself, can often be helpful in allowing an individual to recognize the presence of such existential worries.

Patient Scenario 2

A 45-year-old woman with L-loop single left ventricle, palliated with an atrio-pulmonary Fontan surgery, presents for the third time this year to hospital with intra-atrial reentrant tachycardia, now s/p electrical cardioversion. She has no atrio-ventricular valve regurgitation, no left ventricular outflow obstruction; her left ventricular ejection fraction is 40% on guideline-directed medical therapy, with New York Heart Association functional class IIa, and resting finger pulse oximetry 89%. Computed tomography of the abdomen demonstrates imaging findings consistent with congestive hepatopathy. You are consulted to see her as she feels trapped and uncertain as to how to make a decision about her best next step forward; various consultants have recommended either pharmacotherapy, catheter-based radiofrequency ablation, or surgical Fontan revision with surgical arrhythmia ablation.

Discussion: scenario 2

This short vignette, describing an adult with significant baseline vulnerability to interventions in the setting of preexisting Fontan surgery and recurrent arrhythmia with multiple care options, highlights the nature of complex medical decision-making and attendant personal aspects of risks and benefits; the assistance of an ombudsperson in navigating such may be instrumental in best achieving alignment between patient values, priorities and care choices.

- To an individual patient, for any given intervention, there are
  a. Immediate risks of the action, over hours to days, with short-term, intermediate-term, and long-term uncertainties and consequences, some of which persist or intensify and others of which may be mitigated
  b. Immediate benefits, with similar considerations
  c. Immediate risks of inaction
  d. Benefits and risks that first present in delayed fashion, over weeks to years
  e. Unlikely, yet intense (and potentially intolerable) immediate and delayed risks that have potential to trump other considerations
  f. Benefits that may be critical to meaning-making and life values, which have similar potential to shift prioritization in decision-making.

While review of all of these factors may benefit any and all patients in medicine, such discussion appears even more profound for the ACHD patient with AHD, with complex PPSS factors that contribute to patient values and meaning.

- The ACHD or AHD clinician is experienced and expert in knowledge and practice of data-driven guidelines-directed care management, with recommendations made based upon presenting signs, symptomatology and testing, and recognized aggregate medical outcomes of interventions for a population of similarly affected patients. Patients and families have occasionally commented that such a recommendation tends to "condemn them to live in a world of BEST CASE OUTCOMES," that aligns with statistical best outcomes of relief of shortness of breath, improved exercise capacity, or prolonged survival, though it does not take into account the nuances of real-world occurrences and personal values. To improve relevance of recommendations and to allow for best care-related decision-making that aligns with patient and family priorities, PC clinicians typically present patients with scenarios of what outcomes would realistically look like, from perspectives of not only best-case but also most-likely and worst-case outcomes, inclusive of immediate-term and longer term outcomes. Patients and families recognize how difficult it may be for clinicians to predict outcomes, yet they also acknowledge and rely on the experience that is harbored within such practitioners. Even when data are less robust, clinicians tend to be able to place predictions into categories such as "more (or less) likely than not" or adding "far more (or less)" as qualifiers, when experiential guidance is requested.
- Assessment of external and personal supports for real-world outcomes of interventions (inclusive of assessing adaptive coping skills and assisting in preemptively building such, when deficient) is a well-known and validated component of AHD selection-committees in decision-making regarding candidacy for mechanical circulatory support and transplantation[12]; application of this practice to ACHD patients by PC-experienced clinicians may carry similar import in most appropriate offering of care potentials.

Patient Scenario 3

A 40-year-old man with complete common atrioventricular canal s/p repair and HFpEF presents with marked decline in functional capacity and quality of life (QOL), after recurrent hospitalizations for gastrointestinal bleeding, varices, ammonemia, and associated altered mental status. Between prolonged hospitalizations and extended stays at skilled rehabilitation (due to progressive difficulties emerging from delirium each successive hospitalization), he has spent at most 2 weeks at home over the past 6 months. He has paroxysmal atrial fibrillation, is s/p mitral valve replacement on 3 past occasions, uses oral anticoagulation, has combined group 1 + 2 pulmonary hypertension, and has had renal embolism and postoperative seizures. A decade ago, in the setting of a motorcycle accident, he was recognized to have sustained portal vein thrombosis and subsequent development of cirrhosis. Despite counsel to the contrary, he continued to ride his motorcycle until this year. He consistently described himself as having "joie de vivres." Over the last several hospitalizations, he has shared with you how tormented he has felt not being able to keep control of his thoughts.

Discussion: scenario 3

This short vignette, describing an adult with multiple organ system complications and sequelae of multiple surgeries in the setting of complex congenital heart disease now facing recurrent hospitalizations and progressive decline in critical quality-making and meaning-making aspects of his life, highlights the cardiovascular and noncardiovascular symptom burden and medicalization that can attend the ACHD patient's final year of life.

- In general, ACHD relate similar prevalence of pain, anxiety, depression, and cardiovascular symptomatology when compared to adults with AHD referred for palliative care.[13–15]
- In the last year and months of life, hospitalizations, intensive care unit admissions, 30-day repeat hospital admissions, and length of hospital stay are more frequent for ACHD than for adults with cancer.[16,17]
- Understanding a patient's priorities and values, as well as recognizing the shift in health trajectory that occurs with medical occurrences, allows for prognostic discussions that can help a patient and family recognize that their health and survival are "in a new place," in which reassessing care goals and patient priorities may benefit patient and family in best aligning with care plans. Expressions like "stop fighting," "giving up," and "care withdrawal," despite heartfelt best intention when used, tend to carry derogating connotations; PC clinicians often suggest replacement with transparent terms such as "reprioritizing care goals" to maximize, or protect, priorities. If and when prioritization of care transitions toward focus on symptom mitigation rather than targeting primary-

disease, PC clinicians may be able to aide (with care managers) in navigating such accomplishment either at home or hospital, with home-based palliative care or hospice programs, or general-inpatient hospice when symptoms of burden are in need of acute deintensification.

- Data from oncologic practice (similar to ACHD practice, as noted earlier) suggest that longitudinal subspecialty clinicians understand critical patient goals far less than they believe they do (examples including (a) prioritization of greater time versus quality in life remaining, (b) support from, and strength from religious faith, and (c) of EOL treatments and goals).[18] Having PC-experienced clinicians perform iterative SICs eliciting goals of care and advance care planning has appeared to improve mental health and QOL metrics, as well as decreased resource utilization with similar outcomes, for patients facing EOL with cancer (and in some circumstances, extending time with such improved quality).[19] Given similarities in disease complexity, PPSS stressors and trajectories to EOL, it is anticipated that such PC intervention may have similar patient-centered benefits for ACHD with AHD.

In summary, ACHD clinical care guidelines, position papers, and scientific statements have promulgated access to PC for ACHD, largely based on extrapolation from similarly complex patient populations facing cancer or AHD.[20–22] Interdisciplinary PC teams most typically contain medical physicians, nurse-practitioners (or other advanced practice providers), social workers, and spiritual care consultants, sharing responsibilities toward a common goal of mitigation of suffering. The past decade has witnessed extension of widespread acceptance of embedded palliative care programming in oncologic practice to various care models of PC within AHD programs; it is anticipated that ACHD, as a paradigm of AHD care, will follow suit in incorporating or embedding PC teams within ACHD programming, and hopefully, as a niche subspecialty, will be able to develop robust datasets demonstrating improvement in patient-centered outcomes from such intervention.

CLINICS CARE POINTS

- Assessing risk profiles, ACHD physiologically and clinically appear 20 to 30 years older than their stated age.

- ACHD arry a high burden of cardiac and noncardiac symptomatology, with attendant suffering that comprises components from physical, psychological, social and spiritual domains.
- The potential for impact of embedded palliative care within ACHD programming is highlighted by a) the similar prevalence of pain, anxiety, depression, and cardiovascular symptomatology in ACHD as contrasted to adults with advanced heart disease referred for palliaitve care, and b) the greater relative incidence of hospitalizations, intensive care unit admissions, 30-day repeat hospital admissions, and length of hospital stay, in ACHD as compared to adults with cancer.

DISCLOSURE

None.

REFERENCES

1. Dellborg M, Giang KW, Eriksson P, et al. Circulation. Adults with congenital heart disease: trends in event-free survival past middle age. Circulation 2023;147:930–8.
2. O'Leary JM, Siddiqi OK, de Ferranti S, et al. The changing demographics of congenital heart disease hospitalizations in the United States, 1998 through 2010. JAMA 2013;309:984–6.
3. Van Bulck L, Goossens E, Morin L, et al. BELCODAC consortium. Last year of life of adults with congenital heart diseases: causes of death and patterns of care. Eur Heart J 2022;43:4483–92.
4. Deng LX, Gleason LP, Khan AM, et al. Advance care planning in adults with congenital heart disease: a patient priority. Int J Cardiol 2017;231:105–9.
5. Steiner JM, Kovacs AH. Adults with congenital heart disease: facing morbidities and uncertain early mortality. Prog Pediatr Cardiol 2018;48:75–81.
6. Farr SL, Downing KF, Goudie A, et al. Advance care directives among a population-based sample of young adults with congenital heart defects, CH STRONG, 2016–2019. Pediatr Cardiol 2021;42:1775–84.
7. Steiner JM, Dhami A, Brown CE, et al. Barriers and facilitators of palliative care and advance care planning in adults with congenital heart disease. Am J Cardiol 2020;135:128–34.
8. Steiner JM, Oechslin EN, Veldtman G, et al. Advance care planning and palliative care in ACHD: the healthcare providers' perspective. Cardiol Young 2020;30:402–8.
9. Bolton LE, Seymour J, Gardiner C. Existential suffering in the day to day lives of those living with

palliative care needs arising from chronic obstructive pulmonary disease (COPD): A systematic integrative literature review. Palliat Med 2022;36:567–80.

10. Gillilan R, Qawi S, Weymiller AJ, et al. Spiritual distress and spiritual care in advanced heart failure. Heart Fail Rev 2017;22:581–91.

11. Steinhauser KE, Alexander S, Olsen MK, et al. Addressing patient emotional and existential needs during serious illness: Results of the OUTLOOK randomized controlled trial. J Pain Symptom Manage 2017;54:898–908.

12. Dew MA, Hollenberger JC, Obregon LL, et al. The preimplantation psychosocial evaluation and prediction of clinical outcomes during mechanical circulatory support: what information is most prognostic? Transplantation 2021;105:608–19.

13. Berghammer M, Karlsson J, Ekman I, et al. Self-reported health status (EQ-5D) in adults with congenital heart disease. Int J Cardiol 2013;165:537–43.

14. Kovacs AH, Saidi AS, Kuhl EA, et al. Depression and anxiety in adult congenital heart disease: predictors and prevalence. Int J Cardiol 2009;137:158–64.

15. Warraich HJ, Wolf SP, Mentz RJ, et al. Characteristics and Trends Among Patients With Cardiovascular Disease Referred to Palliative Care. JAMA Netw Open 2019;2:e192375.

16. Tobler D, Greutmann M, Colman JM, et al. End-of-life care in hospitalized adults with complex congenital heart disease: care delayed, care denied. Palliat Med 2012;26:72–9.

17. Steiner JM, Kirkpatrick JN, Heckbert SR, et al. Hospital resource utilization and presence of advance directives at the end of life for adults with congenital heart disease. Congenit Heart Dis 2018;13:721–7.

18. Douglas SL, Daly BJ, Meropol NJ, et al. Patient-physician discordance in goals of care for patients with advanced cancer. Curr Oncol 2019;26:370–9.

19. Bernacki RE, Block SD. American College of Physicians High Value Care Task Force. Communication about serious illness care goals: a review and synthesis of best practices. JAMA Intern Med 2014;174:1994–2003.

20. Stout KK, Daniels CJ, Aboulhosn JA, et al. 2018 AHA/ACC guideline for the management of adults with congenital heart disease: a report of the American College of Cardiology/American Heart Association Task Force on Clinical Practice Guidelines. Circulation 2019;139:e698–800.

21. Schwerzmann M, Goossens E, Gallego P, et al. Recommendations for advance care planning in adults with congenital heart disease: a position paper from the ESC Working Group of Adult Congenital Heart Disease, the Association of Cardiovascular Nursing and Allied Professions (ACNAP), the European Association for Palliative Care (EAPC), and the International Society for Adult Congenital Heart Disease (ISACHD). Eur Heart J 2020;41:4200–10.

22. Blume ED, Kirsch R, Cousino MK, et al. Palliative care across the life span for children with heart disease: A scientific statement from the American Heart Association. Circ Cardiovasc Qual Outcomes 2023;16:e000114.

Special Article

Vision Statement and Call to Action for Adult Congenital Heart Disease Heart Failure

For the last several decades, the majority of those born with congenital heart disease (CHD) have survived to adulthood, and not just those with simple or moderate forms of CHD but also those with complex and severe forms of CHD. The overall prevalence of CHD has shifted to adulthood, driven by the improved survival of those with complex CHD. As such, the median age for patients with complex CHD now sits squarely in adulthood, to be cared for by adult congenital heart disease (ACHD) specialists.[1] And there is no expectation the rise in the number of patients and prevalence of ACHD will slow in near future. Epidemiologic studies have estimated the prevalence of ACHD will continue to rise for the next several decades, possibly doubling by 2050 to 2060.[2,3]

To meet this demand requires a highly specialized, well-trained, and dedicated team to care for the cardiovascular as well the CHD-related noncardiac medical issues. We are, unfortunately, critically behind in the development of sufficient ACHD care models. Despite predications and warnings decades earlier from respected icons and leaders in the field of CHD, we did not begin dedicating resources toward this effort until about a decade ago.[4,5] Today, in the United States, there are approximately one pediatric cardiologist for every 300 patients, and in comparison, one ACHD cardiologist for every 3000 patients. A tenfold difference. Plus, we are not developing sufficient ACHD centers and care teams to meet the needs of the population. The majority of states and geographic regions in the United States have insufficient centers to care for patients with ACHD.[6]

The gap between ACHD population growth and the development of the ACHD services (cardiologists, care teams, subspecialists, centers of excellence) is not narrowing but widening—and will continue to widen until we find ways to bring all stakeholders together and truly dedicate the necessary resources to meet the unique needs of the ACHD population.

A critical part of the ACHD care model is evaluating and treating heart failure (HF). Through large cohort studies, the leading cause of morbidity and mortality for all forms of CHD is HF, particularly affecting the outcome of those with more complex forms of CHD.[7] HF for those with CHD is unique and requires knowledge of both anatomic and physiologic substrates and an understanding of their surgical repair. This is coupled with the effect of the surgical repair on their current state of HF. Those with a systemic right ventricle and with single-ventricle anatomy with Fontan palliation have their own set of unique issues outside of traditional acquired heart disease HF. Uniformly, these two populations will develop HF, and to date, we have limited options especially for those with Fontan palliation outside of heart transplant. The uniqueness of this population and smaller overall numbers have hindered the same progress on several fronts we have witnessed for those with acquired heart disease HF.

Therefore, from the successes of treating pediatric CHD, we have created a "new" population of adults with CHD; they are complex, have a likelihood to develop HF, and are rising at a rate beyond current capacity to provide proper care—and the gap is widening. We are behind in the mechanisms and science leading to the development HF for this population, prevention strategies, risk factor analysis, evaluation tools, and medical and device treatment options, and we are not on the same playing field for transplant consideration as acquired heart disease. Today, every child born with single-ventricle anatomy has a predetermined fate, analogous to a gene defect that uniformly expresses its lethal phenotype later in life. In this case, it's the development of advanced HF, leading to either younger-than-expected CHD-related mortality or, in a smaller percentage, heart or heart-liver transplant. We must change this course, and we must change this trajectory.

Our vision is to align ALL stakeholders, including dedicated individuals, professional and patient advocacy societies, professional board-certifying institutions, training and education bodies, pharmaceutical and medical device companies, national research funding agencies, state and national legislative bodies, and transplant allocation organizations, toward a common goal—to develop strategies, therapies, and research dedicated to better understand ACHD HF, slow the

Heart Failure Clin 20 (2024) 245–247
https://doi.org/10.1016/j.hfc.2024.01.003

rate of ACHD HF, and improve the quality of life and outcome for those with ACHD HF.

CALL TO ACTION

In order to realize this vision and change the course for ACHD HF, recommendations include the following:

- Organizing a multisocietal and stakeholders ACHD HF conference. This would be best developed under the umbrella of a professional organization in cooperation with a patient advocacy society with experience and a track record of success, such as the American College of Cardiology (ACC) and the Adult Congenital Heart Association (ACHA). Invitations to include the following:
  - Subspeciality societies with direct provider and subspecialty impact on ACHD HF
    - American Heart Association
    - ACC's Adult Congenital Pediatric Cardiology Section
    - Heart Failure Society
    - Advanced Cardiac Therapies Improving Network
    - Society of Thoracic Surgery
    - Congenital Heart Surgeons' Society
    - Congenital Heart Public Health Consortium–American Academy of Pediatrics
    - European Society of Cardiology
    - Canadian Cardiology Society
    - Canadian Adult Congenital Heart Network
  - Pharmaceutical and Device Companies with HF therapies
  - Patient advocacy organizations with direct patient impact on ACHD HF
    - ACHA
    - Conquering Congenital Heart Disease
    - Mended Little Hearts
  - Professional Regulatory Organizations with impact on training curriculum and board certification for ACHD HF
    - American Board of Internal Medicine
    - American Board of Pediatrics
    - American Council for Graduate Medical Education
    - American Board of Medical Specialties
  - United Network of Organ Sharing
  - National Research Funding Agencies
    - National Heart, Lung, and Blood Institute
    - Patient-Centered Outcomes and Research Institute
    - American Heart Association

From this stakeholders conference, we would expect collaborative strategies and initiatives to

- Establish an ACHD HF research agenda
- Develop a national ACHD HF patient registry to track patient risk factors and prospective outcomes
- Develop clinical guidelines to highlight gaps in care and assist providers caring for patients with ACHD HF
- Develop feasible training pathways and curriculum to generate highly qualified ACHD HF specialists
- Collect data regarding ACHD transplant to better understand the unique qualifying features of the population (particularly those with single-ventricle Fontan) to improve access to transplant and improve outcomes
- Develop multicenter clinical trials for HF medications and device development for advanced ACHD HF
- Allocate taxpayer resources through legislative efforts for equal support, representation, and access to care, the same as those dedicated to acquired heart disease HF

The ACHD population is growing and outpacing our health care resources. ACHD HF is the most critical issue facing patients, providers, and ACHD care teams. We are behind in our efforts, and the gap is widening. Yet, we have the expertise, the drive, the potential resources, and the willingness to change this course. The complexity of the ACHD HF requires a complex solution of multisocietal and *patient advocacy-driven* collaboration. With this, we can realize the vision of improved care and outcomes for those with ACHD HF.

Curt J. Daniels, MD
Columbus Ohio Adult
Congenital Heart Program
Department of Internal Medicine and Pediatrics
The Ohio State University and
Nationwide Children's Hospital
473 West 12th Avenue, Suite 200
Columbus, OH 43210, USA

E-mail address:
Curt.Daniels@osumc.edu

REFERENCES

1. Marelli AJ, Ionescu-Ittu R, Mackie AS, et al. Lifetime prevalence of congenital heart disease in the general population from 2000 to 2010. Circulation 2014;130(9):749–56.
2. Baumgartner H. Geriatric congenital heart disease: a new challenge in the care of adults with congenital heart disease? Eur Heart J 2014;35(11):683–5.
3. Benziger CP, Stout K, Zaragoza-Macias E, et al. Projected growth of the adult congenital heart disease

population in the United States to 2050: an integrative systems modeling approach. Popul Health Metr 2015; 13:29.

4. Perloff JK. Congenital heart disease in adults. A new cardiovascular subspecialty. Circulation 1991;84(5): 1881–90.

5. Somerville J. Congenital heart disease in adults and adolescents. Br Heart J 1986;56(5): 395–7.

6. Fernandes SM, Marelli A, Hile DM, et al. Access and delivery of adult congenital heart disease care in the United States: quality-driven team-based care. Cardiol Clin 2020;38(3):295–304.

7. Diller GP, Kempny A, Alonso-Gonzalez R, et al. Survival prospects and circumstances of death in contemporary adult congenital heart disease patients under follow-up at a large tertiary centre. Circulation 2015;132(22): 2118–25.

Moving?

Make sure your subscription moves with you!

To notify us of your new address, find your **Clinics Account Number** (located on your mailing label above your name), and contact customer service at:

Email: journalscustomerservice-usa@elsevier.com

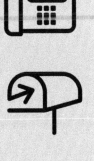

800-654-2452 (subscribers in the U.S. & Canada)
314-447-8871 (subscribers outside of the U.S. & Canada)

Fax number: 314-447-8029

Elsevier Health Sciences Division
Subscription Customer Service
3251 Riverport Lane
Maryland Heights, MO 63043

Printed and bound by CPI Group (UK) Ltd, Croydon, CR0 4YY

03/10/2024

01040365-0011